Monalisa C. M. Silva
Edna A. B. Castro

Elderly people caring for an elderly relative at home:

Monalisa C. M. Silva
Edna A. B. Castro

Elderly people caring for an elderly relative at home:

Religiosity/Spirituality as a relief from tensions

ScienciaScripts

Imprint

Any brand names and product names mentioned in this book are subject to trademark, brand or patent protection and are trademarks or registered trademarks of their respective holders. The use of brand names, product names, common names, trade names, product descriptions etc. even without a particular marking in this work is in no way to be construed to mean that such names may be regarded as unrestricted in respect of trademark and brand protection legislation and could thus be used by anyone.

Cover image: www.ingimage.com

This book is a translation from the original published under ISBN 978-613-9-62096-8.

Publisher:
Sciencia Scripts
is a trademark of
Dodo Books Indian Ocean Ltd. and OmniScriptum S.R.L publishing group

120 High Road, East Finchley, London, N2 9ED, United Kingdom
Str. Armeneasca 28/1, office 1, Chisinau MD-2012, Republic of Moldova, Europe
Printed at: see last page
ISBN: 978-620-7-71308-0

SUMMARY

ACKNOWLEDGMENTS

The meaning of THANKSGIVING lies in the possibility of recognizing that, in our existence here on earth, we will be able to evolve if we are allowed to count on the sublime cooperation of our family members, teachers, colleagues and friends, being permeated by the superior energy that surrounds our being. For this, I report and thank you:

To GOD, my father, eternal protector, the One who created us, the reason for my existence. Who, every day, invites me to live his LOVE, his MERCY, his FORGIVENESS, and invites me to be a temple of the Holy Spirit. Thank you, my Lord, for welcoming me into your arms and offering me boundless love. Thank you, my father, for giving me the strength and patience to wait for the right time to complete my master's degree (and how I waited); and for giving me the wisdom to overcome all the obstacles in my life and on the paths of research and teaching.

TO MY PARENTS, for being my foundation, my safe haven. I thank them for their full-time dedication to my children, especially Ana Clara, who is only two years old. Especially my mother, who has always been by my side, in the days and nights of anguish, always making me realize that this is only the beginning of my victories on this path that I have been walking with love and dedication.

TO MY HUSBAND, my partner, who came into my life like a Godsend. Thank you for your understanding of my absence as a wife and companion at times when I was studying, reading, researching; and how many early mornings and weekends were like that... Thank you for your support and for the many times you took care of Ana Clara on Saturdays and Sundays. Thank you for being part of our lives.

TO MY CHILDREN, Gabriel and Ana Clara. As I always say: you are my life, my light, witnesses to God's love in my life. Gabriel, my prince, a special child, an angel in my life, thank you for your understanding in the many moments when I was stressed, with so many things to study. You teach me a lot and make me grow every day. Ana Clara, so small and yet so important in my life, you can't imagine how much good it does me when I get home and you run into my arms with your little eyes shining with happiness and start shouting: "Mama!". I will thank God every day of my life for allowing me such happiness: to be a MOTHER. I LOVE YOU.

TO MY DEAR GRANDMA, Eliodora, who is no longer with us, but has always kept me in her prayers, and I believe she continues to watch over me. And to my uncle, Celso, who gave up his life to care for her until the last moment of her life, with total dedication and love.

When I was researching family caregivers, I felt all the burden that was on them and often, unfortunately, I couldn't help them as I should have. Thank you always.

TO MY FRIEND and comrade-in-law Nirema, who was always there, encouraging and collaborating in every possible way. Thank you, my friend, for everything you do for me and my children, for your prayers and for always being willing to help.

To Prof.[a] Dr. EDNA, my advisor, for all her attention and for enriching this work. Thank you from the bottom of my heart for believing in me when I needed it most. In a moment of anguish and sadness, when so many doors closed, you accepted me and welcomed me into your research group, GAPESE, where I quickly matured my ideas, my thoughts, which led me to reflect on the life of the caregiver who is already elderly. Within a few meetings, I had already found my object of study. I sincerely thank you for allowing me to complete such an important stage in my life, supporting and encouraging me to move forward with what I believed in. I'm sure I'll be eternally grateful for everything you've done for me.

To the PROFESSORS: Dr. Bruno David Henriques, Dr. Alexander Moreira-Almeida, Dr. Sonia Maria Soares and Dr. Sônia Maria Dias, who so kindly agreed to sit on my examining board and for their rich contributions to this study.

To the Faculty of Nursing of the Federal University of Juiz de Fora (UFJF), for giving me the opportunity to study for a master's degree, contributing to my professional growth.

To the coordinator of the Master's in Nursing at UFJF, Dr. Anna Maria de Oliveira Salimena, for her dedication, her concern at all times and for the excellent work she has done.

To all the teachers in the Department of Basic Nursing, for their support and understanding during the difficult moments of this journey.

To all the teachers who took part in this master's degree, for their teachings, which I will carry with me throughout my professional life.

To the secretariat of the Master's in Nursing at UFJF, especially Elisângela Trovato, who was always dedicated and attended to us promptly at all times.

To all the members of the Study and Research Group on Self-Care and the Educational Process in Health and Nursing (GAPESE), who directly or indirectly accompanied me during this journey, especially Camila Medeiros, Irene Duarte, and fellow master's students Denicy Chagas and Denise Rocha. Thank you for the moments of learning and for being able to share guidance and the development of so much work together.

To my colleagues at the Spirituality and Health Research Center (NUPES), who, despite the short time we've been together, have contributed to my professional and personal growth at every meeting and to the completion of this work through the sharing of knowledge at each meeting.

To the Community Health Agents I met during the course of this research, who welcomed and accompanied me with such respect and generosity and, at every visit, opened the way for my arrival.

To all the elderly (caregivers and people being cared for) and to my uncle who, although not yet elderly, took care of my dear grandmother for many years, I dedicate this work to you, which I did with great love and dedication. I thank you for having awakened even more in me the desire to be close to you, to study everything that permeates the health of the elderly and, above all, spirituality. I thank you for opening your homes to me with such affection and availability, for sharing your memories and experiences, of happy moments and sad ones, for enriching my study with such WISDOM AND SIMPLICITY. You have taught me to love more, to care better, to overcome difficulties and never give up and, above all, you have shown me that without the most important thing, without spiritual strength, nothing is possible. After all, we are energy, we are spiritual beings. So we have to have faith and hope in what we can't see, because the moment we try to spiritualize ourselves, we can feel it; and how magnificent that feeling is! May I one day be able to reciprocate with the same hug, smile and sparkle in the eyes of those people who, even with so much responsibility to take care of a person in their entirety, have offered me affection in every encounter.

EPIGRAFE

"Throughout our lives there are clues that point us in the right direction. If we don't pay attention to these clues, we make the wrong choices and end up living an unhappy life. If we pay attention, we learn our lessons and have a full and good life, as well as a good death. The greatest gift God has given us is free will. Free will puts the responsibility for making the best possible choices on our shoulders."

(Kubler-Ross, 1998).

SUMMARY

Introduction: The process of demographic and epidemiological transition, followed by the progressive increase in the number of elderly people, points to a new reality: the need for elderly family caregivers. **Objective: To** analyze the elements that make up the process of caring for an elderly person at home, by a family member who is also elderly. **Methods:** Qualitative research based on Grounded Theory, carried out in the municipality of Juiz de Fora, Minas Gerais. Data collection took place between August 2014 and January 2015, with ten elderly caregivers participating in the study. In the seventh interview, it was observed that the participants' answers had become redundant and it was not relevant to continue with the data collection. However, as a way of validating the theory, we returned to the field for another three interviews, in order to allow for a deeper and richer systematic comparative analysis and interpretation of the data. During this phase, we sought out caregivers with different socio-economic levels in order to better understand their experiences. Home visits were used for data collection, with interviews, observation and recording of notes in a field diary, as well as the preparation of memos. The OpenLogos® program was used for textual editing and coding of the empirical data. **Results:** Forty codes emerged from the data, which made up four categories: "Aging and becoming a family caregiver"; "Family support"; "The elderly caregiver who cares daily for an elderly person at home and the health team"; and "The spiritual dimension influencing the life and care process of an elderly family caregiver", which was the central category of the study. The central category allowed us to understand how elderly family caregivers experience the process of caring for an elderly family member at home, even in the face of negative repercussions, such as the lack of family support, and the difficulties experienced in everyday life, such as the lack of institutionalized support for caring for others. Regardless of whether or not they have family or institutional support, caregivers find empowerment to face the challenges of being a family caregiver on a daily basis through religiosity/spirituality. At this stage of life, there is a change in perspective from a materialistic and pragmatic view of the world to a cosmic and transcendent one. While they seek support from a metaphysical force, the participants use spiritual religious c *oping,* which are the strategies they use to cope with the situations that arise in their lives, attributing to the sacred the strength to persevere and continue along their path, growing old and caring for one or more people, also elderly, at home. **Conclusion:** The religiosity/spirituality of the elderly caregiver proved to be an important strategy used as a support for life's adversities. It is recommended that the spiritual dimension should be considered as an element to assist in the health care process, given that spirituality is accentuated at this stage of life, as the elderly are introspective, rethinking and evaluating their entire lives. The findings reinforce the need for public policies to care for the family caregiver of the elderly, especially the elderly who care for another elderly person at home. As a contribution to the field of practice, this study reinforces the importance of making spirituality a cross-cutting theme in the training curricula of health professionals.

Keywords: Caregivers. Elderly. Spirituality. Home care. Nursing.

THE PATHS THAT BROUGHT ME HERE

Although no one can go back and make a new beginning, anyone can start now and make a new end.

Chico Xavier

The special concern for others has been consolidated in my life trajectory, even before my academic experience. From a very young age, I empirically developed the skills to care for the people around me, which is why I was called upon when someone in the neighborhood fell ill and even to help prepare the bodies of elderly neighbors who died. I started a degree in nursing at the Federal University of Juiz de Fora (UFJF) in 1996 and, after completing the course, I began my professional life in Juiz de Fora, where I worked for a few months in psychiatry, which only confirmed for me that, in order to provide comprehensive care, it is not necessary to detach oneself from the spiritual dimension, because, in order to care, we need to be with the other.

In 2001, I moved to a city in Acre, Cruzeiro do Sul, which is in the northern region of Brazil, located in the far west of the country, bordering Peru. I lived there for ten years, combining my personal life with nursing work, in direct patient care, in a General Hospital and Maternity Hospital of the National Health Foundation (FUNASA). Working as a consultant for UNESCO and in the area of Collective Health, in the Family Health Strategy (ESF), was a great professional experience, because working in the ESF is undoubtedly brilliant. We discovered that we were part of the daily lives of people who, until then, we had only known in a health situation in a hospital. Working in the ESF, we began to enter people's homes, get to know their daily lives and understand them, in this context, as beings of extreme relevance to the health care process. During my daily home visits, I began to realize that elderly people were looking after other elderly people on their own and, in my opinion, this was not an easy task.

I'm at a loss for words to explain what it was like to work in the Amazon region: it was a period of intense learning, in a place with diverse cultures that blended naturally. From then on, I was able to experience different things, working with rural, riverside and indigenous communities. What a wealth! How much I learned from those people!

The importance of perceiving others through their biopsychosocial and spiritual dimensions has always been present in my professional life, because I have never been able to conceive of health care without looking at the individuality of each person who has passed through my hands, with their cultural and creedal differences. The clientele itself, with its accentuated cultural diversity, has helped me to learn, every day, the importance of seeing the other person as a unique being, with their individualities and beliefs, and that these must be respected by health professionals.

In 2009, the course of my life was changed by a competitive examination I took at the Federal University of Acre, when I left direct patient care and took on the role of lecturer at the Federal University of Acre. Still in my infancy, with only a few months of teaching under my belt, I returned to my hometown, now as a teacher in the higher education career, at the Federal University of Juiz de Fora, in the Faculty of Nursing (FACENF). As soon as I arrived, I was assigned to the Departments of Basic Nursing and Applied Nursing, where I taught practical and theoretical classes in the subject of Mental Health, where I had the opportunity to create a Mental Health practice group in Primary Care, a field that could show students the importance of working on mental health, regardless of the area of activity. In the other department, I started with practical classes in Fundamentals of Nursing II and Nursing Administration I and II.

How many changes in such a short space of time. Until then, I didn't really know the size of the responsibility I was taking on. I soon began to realize how hard I had to work to train myself. Then the struggle began, with difficulties in understanding English better and in conceiving the pre-project. After all, until then, I was unfamiliar with academic life and research, as I was part of the last nursing class at UFJF that didn't have to do the Final Project.

There have been many clashes, many struggles, sometimes internal; many times I've thought about giving up because of the external and internal pressure I've been under. But anyway, I'm here now and, of course, I'm persistent, I'm firmly pursuing my goals. In the beginning it was difficult, I couldn't even find something that could be the subject of my research which, as I've been learning, would have to be something that motivated me, because a researcher must be motivated by a restlessness that makes him overcome any difficulty in order to achieve his goal.

After two attempts at selection in another Postgraduate Program, in which I took part up to the interview stage, but was unsuccessful, I joined the Study and Research Group on Self-Care and the Educational Process in Health and Nursing (GAPESE) in 2012. It was then that I became particularly interested in the field of gerontology, but I was still unable to define an object of study. My difficulty was made all the greater by the fact that I am very easy to adapt to, which means that I have several areas of interest.

During a meeting of the research group, after discussing the process of self-care for patients after hospital discharge, I began to imagine what life would be like for a caregiver who is elderly and is responsible for caring for another elderly person. From then on, I began to establish a bridge with my daily practice as a care nurse in the north of Brazil, when I worked in the Family Health Strategy (ESF). When I made home visits to families in my area of work, I noticed that many elderly people had an elderly relative as their main caregiver, who were usually spouses or partners and daughters who, in turn, also lived with health problems, causing a certain degree of difficulty in caring for others and themselves. These caregivers were unprepared to look after a dependent elderly relative at home, as well as to look after themselves. Most of them expressed comfort when their loved one was hospitalized, reporting that this way they shared the care tasks with the nursing team and, above all, they didn't feel so alone and vulnerable.

Currently, during my time as a nursing teacher in the Department of Basic Nursing, in the subject of Fundamentals of Nursing II, and also in an Extension Project focusing on the health of the elderly in Primary Health Care (PHC), I was able to asystematically observe the same situations, which began to provoke concerns, arousing my interest in understanding how elderly people, who care for an elderly relative at home, carry out self-care, how they seek relief from the tensions of everyday life? How do they feel in their daily lives with the responsibility of caring for others? In addition to this question, others arise: do they receive home visits from the ESF nurse? Do they receive institutionalized nursing support for their care tasks? How do they solve their health care needs when their physical and emotional capacity for self-care is exhausted?

One assumption is that, in order to perform well in caring for the elderly, health professionals, supported by a health policy, must offer guidance, support and education, according to the needs and demands of the caregivers and the elderly people they care for. Self-care becomes a goal, especially from a therapeutic perspective, when the family's relationship with the health-disease-care process is fragile, which shows real demands to follow a prescribed treatment. Another assumption is that nursing care needs to extend to the caregiver, based on the premise that the activity of caring for a dependent elderly person generates wear and tension, leading to impairment of the caregiver's physical, mental and social health.

1. INTRODUCTION

True wealth is the wealth of the spirit based on generosity, selflessness, dedicated love, with the awareness that you are fulfilling your life's mission.

Leocàdio José Correia

This research focuses on the process of caring for an elderly person by a family member who is also elderly, at home.

The last half of the 20th century saw a demographic transition, now understood as the longevity revolution, in which more people are living much longer (Butler, 2008). According to data from the United Nations (2012), there were around 810 million people aged 60 or over in the world, and this number is expected to grow to more than 2 billion by 2050. This will be when, for the first time in history, the elderly will outnumber children (0-14 years). Asia has more than half (55%) of the world's older people, followed by Europe with 21%. The data also shows that, although the ageing process is evolving rapidly in developed countries, less developed regions will also experience the same transition process rapidly, in a short period of time (UNITED NATIONS, 2012).

The world is going through a historic process of demographic transition which is being helped by the reduction in birth and death rates, resulting in older populations all over the world. By 2050, one in five people will be aged 60 or over. Faced with this phenomenon, the global community has recognized the need to integrate the process of global ageing into a broader context of development and to design policies based on a longer "life course" and a broader societal perspective. The idea is to create a new image for ageing and convey it to the world stage through ageing policies (UNITED NATIONS, 2014).

The 2010 age pyramids of the Brazilian Institute of Geography and Statistics (IBGE) show an increase in the number of elderly people in Brazil, which will continue to rise in the coming years. Thus, the representation of the population in 1980 was triangular in shape, with a broad base and a narrow peak. This changed in 2010 and will continue to change, according to projections for 2050, when it will no longer be triangular in shape. According to the IBGE age pyramids, seen in Figures 1, 2 and 3, Brazilian population projections can be compared at three different times, retrospectively and prospectively (IBGE, 2013):

Figure 1: Brazilian age pyramid in 1980

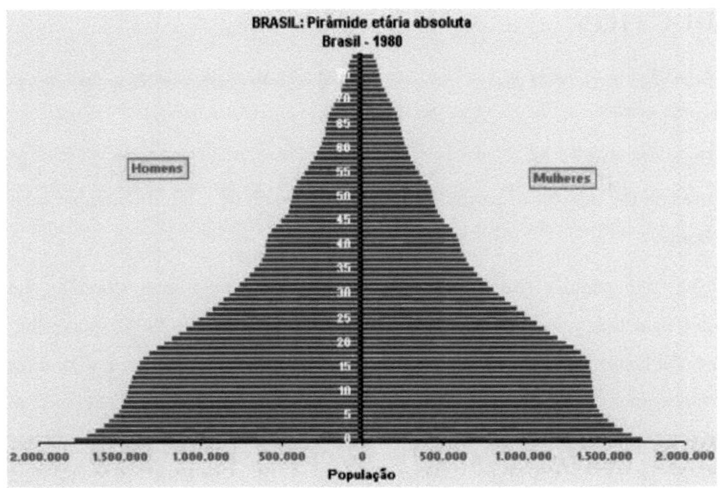

Source: Brazilian Institute of Geography and Statistics

Figure 2: Brazilian age pyramid in 2010

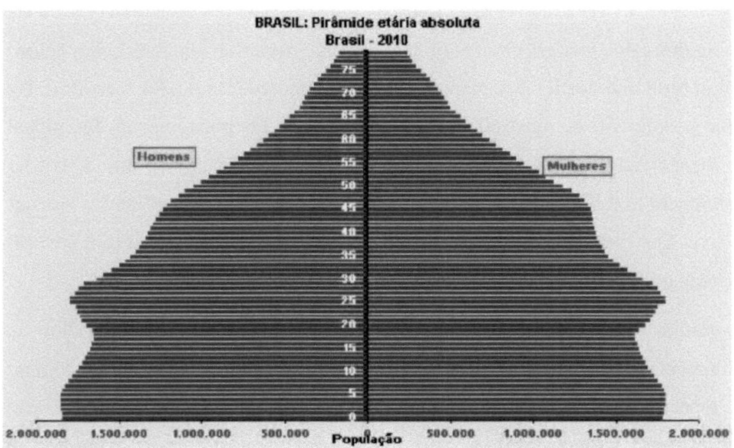

Source: Brazilian Institute of Geography and Statistics

Figure 3: Brazilian age pyramid for the year 2050

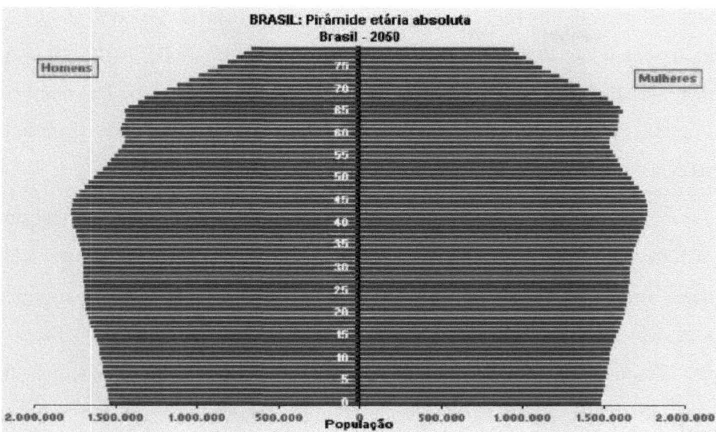

Source: Brazilian Institute of Geography and Statistics

For Vasconcelos and Gomes (2012), the demographic transition process in Brazil can be explained by the occurrence of some phenomena from 1950 onwards: falls in mortality, birth rates and fertility, thus characterizing the increase in life expectancy and survival at advanced ages, which, according to Gonzaga (2014), is related to advances in the health area, as well as investment in sanitation and education.

Analogous to the phenomenon of demographic transition is the process of epidemiological transition in the country, when infectious diseases are controlled by vaccines, drugs and sanitation measures, reducing the incidence of diseases, including chronic non-communicable diseases, whose external causes have become prevalent, mainly affecting the elderly population (CHAIMOWICZ, 2013).

An analysis of IBGE (2010a) data also shows that the ageing index is a "marker" for changes in the age composition of the Brazilian population. In 2010, for every 100 children aged 0 to 14, there were approximately 31 elderly people aged 65 or over. By 2050, the expectation is that the picture will change and, for every 100 children aged 0 to 14, there will be approximately 172 elderly people. An important figure, according to the IBGE (2008), refers to the Southeast region, where there are approximately 9.4 million elderly people, 2.2 million of them in Minas Gerais (IBGE, 2009).

In the municipality of Juiz de Fora - Minas Gerais (MG), the situation is no different from the global population profile, following the world trend, with a slowdown in the growth rate and an evolution of the age pyramid in the older age groups. According to IBGE figures, 13.7% of Juiz de Fora's population is aged 60 or over (IBGE, 2010b). Drawing a parallel with

Uberlândia-MG, which has a slightly higher number of inhabitants than Juiz de Fora, 604,013, the latter overtakes it, which has 12.4% of its citizens aged 60 or over (IBGE, 2010c). It also has a higher average than the state of Minas Gerais with 11.9% (IBGE, 2010d). The number of elderly people in Juiz de Fora also exceeds the national percentage: the elderly represent 20,566,363 of Brazilians, totaling 11% of the population (IBGE, 2010e).

Chaimowicz (2013) analyzes the fact that Brazil is heading for an age revolution and that, in 25 years' time, it will have the title of "ageing country", with child mortality under control and epidemics of dengue fever and yellow fever, while at the same time being increasingly affected by cases of depression in the elderly, Parkinson's disease and Alzheimer's disease. This is why aging can be conceptualized as a natural and progressive process, which distinguishes a stage of life made up of various alterations: physical, mental and social, resulting from the natural wear and tear of bodily, psychological and cognitive structures (FRIES; PEREIRA, 2011).

There is a chasm between practice and discourse on hierarchical models of complexity, with the aim of providing comprehensive care for all elderly people. And, for the authors, age itself becomes the main risk factor for most of the diseases that affect the elderly (VERAS; CALDAS, 2004). One study points out that "chronic conditions" encompass an extremely broad category of ailments that offer common points: they are persistent and require a certain level of permanent care, requiring changes in lifestyle and health management (CARREIRA; RODRIGUES, 2010).

As a result of the various problems that can affect health and, above all, without monitoring, the individual can develop functional incapacity, which can be conceptualized as a difficulty or the need for help for the individual to carry out basic activities of daily living (BADL); or even instrumental activities of daily living (IADL), which are essential for independent living in the community, such as tasks related to mobility (ALVES; LEITE; MACHADO, 2008, 2010; FREITAS et al., 2012; BARBOSA et al., 2014)

According to the aforementioned authors, BADLs consist of self-care tasks, such as bathing, dressing, eating, lying down in/getting out of bed, using the toilet, walking from one room to another, which are often used as indicators of functional incapacity; and IADLs are adaptive or indispensable tasks for independent living in society, for example: shopping, telephoning, using transportation, doing household chores, preparing a meal, managing one's own money (ALVES; LEITE; MACHADO, 2008; FREITAS et al., 2012; BARBOSA et al., 2014).

According to Santos (2014), elderly people go through various transformations as they get older, and when they are diagnosed with a chronic illness, they can enter a stage of imbalance, which must be explained from a constructive perspective by health professionals. In addition, over the years and as a result of the progressive growth in the number of elderly people, the role of caregiver has been revived, since it is the caregiver who, in the home, carries out or helps the elderly person to carry out their activities of daily living (ADL) and instrumental activities of daily living (IADL), with the aim of preserving their autonomy and independence (MAZZA; LÈFEVRE, 2005; VIEIRA et al., 2011).

This research is justified in view of the urgent need for the fields of health policy, planning and politics to turn their attention to the family, especially those who share the burden of health care with the state.

Care for the elderly is one of the focuses of the ESF and, as *already* mentioned, it is important to extend this to their caregivers. To this end, the team's professionals must be prepared with the skills required for the health care required by home care, contributing to the achievement of the objectives set by the National Health Policy for the Elderly (PNSPI), which is the current challenge for the Teams.

1.1 NATIONAL AGENDA OF HEALTH RESEARCH PRIORITIES

Currently, research in the area of care for the elderly is included as a priority for the Ministry of Health (FERNANDES; SOARES, 2012). As it is considered a phenomenon of global proportions, the subject of population ageing is dealt with on a recurring basis in various countries, including Brazil, since the subject gives rise to relevant allusions at social and economic levels to the lives of the population and to public coffers (CHAIMOWICZ, 2013).

This gave rise to the construction and implementation of the National Agenda for Health Research Priorities, which is "a political process that seeks, in all its stages, the broad participation of actors with different experiences and languages in both research and health" (BRASIL, 2008a, P. 5). The National Agenda for Health Research Priorities is based on the assumption that it "respects national and regional health needs and increases selective induction for the production of knowledge and material and procedural goods in priority areas for the development of social policies" (Brasil, 2008a, p. 13). This agenda was established as the first exercise in defining health research priorities in Brazil.

The discussion around the Agenda is a relevant action to legitimize this instrument in the National Policy for Science, Technology and Innovation in Health, allowing health research priorities to be in line with the principles of the SUS. Its assumptions are based on national and regional health needs, as well as the aim of broadening selective induction for the production of knowledge in priority areas for the development of social policies (BRASIL,

2008a).

The importance of studying ageing stems from the need to carry out research in a field in which, until now, there has been little mastery and knowledge. Its approach in primary health care is centered on the socio-political interface with health care, whose research has been developed in isolation, this being one of the topics that generates the most interest, due to the growing demand from the ageing population (FERNANDES; SOARES, 2012).

Thus, studies and research centered on nursing, focusing on both the elderly and caregivers, especially informal caregivers, are becoming increasingly important, given the context of aging and increased demands for home care in which we live. The topic in question is included in the priorities of the Elderly Health area, in the National Research Agenda, under item "6.1.2.1 Studies on the role of the elderly as caregivers" (BRASIL, 2008a, p.19).

This study is relevant because of the need to provide a basis for primary health care, which plays an essential role in maintaining continuity of care for the elderly and their caregivers, who are also elderly, linked to home care. It is necessary to gather the subjects' point of view on their needs and demands, within the scope of this new type of care, in accordance with what has potential for the evolution of health practice and, in particular, nursing practice.

We hope to contribute to building knowledge about the care needs demanded by elderly users who care for other elderly people at home, with a view to strengthening health promotion work, prioritized by SUS legislation, as well as being in line with the principles of universal and comprehensive care. Thus, when we refer to the integrality of care, we cannot fail to highlight that the spiritual dimension is intrinsic to the human being, recognizable when it arises as a need and, therefore, inherent in nursing care. However, nurses show insecurity and subjectivity when defining so-called subjective concepts, such as the spiritual dimension, so much so that they insist on suppressing it, most of the time, during the care they provide.

It is believed that by investing in this research, as well as in disseminating its findings, scientific discourse will be given greater visibility and, consequently, the reliability of practices will be guaranteed. From this perspective, we believe that the research could contribute to the knowledge and integration of various dimensions in the practice of health teams, with an emphasis on nursing care.

2. OBJECTIVES

2.1 GENERAL:

To analyze the elements that make up the process of caring for an elderly person at home by a family member who is also elderly.

2.2 SPECIFIC:

• To analyze how elderly people who take care of an elderly relative take care of themselves;

• Identify the strategies used by caregivers to relieve the tensions related to the caregiving process;

• Observing the facilities and difficulties elderly caregivers have in caring for their family members on a daily basis;

• Developing a theoretical flowchart on the process of care at home for elderly people caring for an elderly relative.

3. THEORETICAL FRAMEWORK

Everything that exists and lives needs to be cared for in order to continue to exist. A plant, a child, an elderly person, planet Earth. Everything that lives needs to be fed. So care, the essence of human life, needs to be continually nurtured. Care thrives on love, tenderness, affection and coexistence.

Leonardo Boff, 1999

3.1 ELDERLY CARE POLICY

According to the World Health Organization (WHO), an elderly person is considered to be 60 years of age or older if they live in developing countries, and this limit becomes 65 years of age in developed countries (WORLD HEALTH ORGANIZATION, 1984). In Brazil, the Statute of the Elderly (BRASIL, 2003) followed the same chronological age criterion, defining the elderly as those aged 60 or over.

A preliminary review of the literature on Brazilian legislation concerning people aged 60 and over shows that the aging process in Brazil, from a legal perspective, includes Law No. 8,842, which provides for the National Elderly Health Policy (PNSI), having been enacted in 1994 and regulated in 1996, by means of Decree 1,948/1996, of July 3, 1996. The law ensured social rights for the elderly, creating conditions to promote their autonomy, integration and effective participation in society, reaffirming their right to health at the various levels of SUS care (BRASIL, 2010). Its main objective was to create favorable conditions for longevity with quality of life.

In 1999, Ordinance No. 1.395/GM of December 10, 1999 was promulgated, approving the proposal for a policy on the health of the elderly by the Tripartite Interagency Commission and the National Health Council, on the National Policy on the Health of the Elderly (BRASIL, 1999). As mentioned in the previous ordinance, the return to the home care model, which has been widely discussed, cannot be aimed solely at reducing costs or even transferring responsibilities. Home care for the elderly, whose functional capacity is compromised, requires guidance programs, information and advice from specialists (BRASIL, 1999).

In 2002, the organization and implementation of state networks for the care of the elderly was proposed (Ordinance No. 702/SAS/MS, 2002), based on the management conditions and division of responsibilities defined by the Operational Standard for Health Care (NOAS). As part of the operationalization of the networks, rules were created for the registration of reference centers for elderly health care (BRASIL, 2006a).

Law 10.741, of October 1, 2003, which provides for the Statute of the Elderly, was approved and sanctioned, expanding the response of the state and society to the needs of the elderly population, but it did not provide the means to finance the proposed actions. Chapter IV focused specifically on the role of the SUS in providing comprehensive health care for the elderly, guaranteeing universal and equal access, in an articulated and continuous set of actions and services, for the prevention, promotion, protection and recovery of health, including special attention to diseases that preferentially affect the elderly (BRASIL, 2003). The entry into force of the Statute and its use as an instrument for winning the rights of the elderly and expanding the ESF revealed the presence of elderly people and fragile families, in situations of social vulnerability and the still incipient insertion of state networks to assist the health of the elderly, making it essential to readjust the PNSI (BRASIL, 2006a).

In February 2006, Ordinance No. 399/GM, of February 22, 2006, published the Pact for Health Guidelines, covering the Pact for Life. In this document, the health of the elderly came to be seen as one of the six priorities agreed upon by the three spheres of government, and a series of actions were proposed which ultimately aimed to implement some of the guidelines, one of which was the National Health Policy for the Elderly (PNSPI) (BRASIL, 2006b). In the light of the above, Ministerial Order GM/MS No. 2.528 of October 19, 2006 was issued, approving the National Health Policy for Older People (PNSPI), with the main purpose of:

"to recover, maintain and promote the autonomy and independence of elderly individuals, directing collective and individual health measures to this end, in line with the principles and guidelines of the Unified Health System (SUS). This policy is aimed at all Brazilian citizens aged 60 or over" (BRASIL, 2006a p. 3).

3.2 PRIMARY HEALTH CARE (PHC) AND THE FAMILY HEALTH STRATEGY (ESF)

The first definition of Primary Health Care (PHC) was proposed at the "International Conference on Primary Health Care" in the city of Alma-Ata, Kazakhstan, in the former Soviet Union, in 1978, when they proposed an agreement and a goal among its member countries to achieve the highest possible level of health by the year 2000. This international policy became known as "Health for All by the Year 2000". The Alma-Ata Declaration, as the agreement signed by 134 countries was called, advocated the following definition of PHC, here referred to as primary health care:

Primary health care is essential health care based on practical, scientifically well-founded and socially acceptable methods and technologies, made universally available to individuals and families in the community, through their full participation and at a cost that the community and the country can afford at every stage of its development, in the spirit of self-reliance and self-medication. They are an integral part of both the country's health system, of which they are the central function and main focus, and the community's overall social and economic development. They represent the first level of contact between the individual, the family and the community and the national health system, through which health care is brought as close as possible to the places where people live and work, and constitute the first element of a continuous process of health care (DE ALMA ATA, 1978).

Soon, various definitions of PHC began to emerge. For Starfield, a researcher in primary health care and a reference for the Ministry of Health, PHC forms the basis that will define the work at the other levels of access to the health system, leading to the organization and rationalization of the use of resources, both basic and specialized, aimed at health promotion, prevention and recovery (STARFIELD, 2004). Thus, PHC is the level of the health system which, preferably, will be the gateway to the user's needs and problems and which should provide care for the person and not just for the illness, over time and for all conditions.

According to Gomes *et al.* (2011), according to the Alma-Ata Declaration, PHC comprises, among other proposals, the main health care, which should be based on accessible technologies, so that it can bring health services as close as possible to the places where people live and work, thus making up the first level of contact with the national health system and the first element of a continuous process of care.

In this sense, the need arose to create universal health systems, i.e. that conceive of health as a human right and, in the 80s of the 20th century, the understanding that health is the result of economic and social conditions, as well as inequalities between different countries; it also stipulates that national governments should promote the management of health systems, stimulating exchange and international technological, economic and political support (MATTA, 2005).

From then on, there were rudimentary PHC experiments in Brazil from the beginning of the 20th century, culminating in the health movement, when PHC concepts were incorporated into the reformist ideology, including the need to reorient the current care model, thus breaking with the privatized medical model centered on the individual, which was in force until the beginning of the 80s. There were countless experiences which, together with the constitution of the SUS (Brazil, 1988) and its regulation (Brazil, 1990), made it possible to build a Primary Health Care (PHC) policy that tended to reorient the care model, giving rise to a priority relationship between the population and the health system (LAVRAS, 2011).

There have been several moves to strengthen PHC in the country, including the creation of the Department of Primary Care (DAB) by the Ministry of Health in 2000, the implementation of the National Primary Care Policy (PNAB) and the Pact for Health and Life, in 2006, documents that reiterated, with primacy, the consolidation and qualification of the Family

Health Strategy as a PHC model and the organizing center of health care networks (GOMES *et al.*, 2011). In this way, the understanding of PHC developed from the principles of the SUS, especially universality, decentralization, integrality and popular participation, as can be seen in the ordinance establishing the PNAB, which defines PHC as:

A set of health actions in the individual and collective spheres that encompass health promotion and protection, disease prevention, diagnosis, treatment, rehabilitation and health maintenance. It is developed through the exercise of democratic and participatory management and health practices, in the form of teamwork, directed at populations in well-defined territories, for which they assume health responsibility, taking into account the dynamics existing in the territory in which these populations live. It uses high-complexity, low-density technologies to solve the most frequent and relevant health problems in its territory. It is the users' preferred contact with health systems. It is guided by the principles of universality, accessibility and coordination of care, linkage and continuity, comprehensiveness, accountability, humanization, equity and social participation (Brazil, 2011a).

Currently, the main PHC strategy in Brazil is family health, which has been receiving financial incentives with the aim of expanding population coverage and reorganizing care. The ESF was originally conceived as the Family Health Program (PSF) in 1994, strongly linked to the situation of communities, and was initially implemented in small towns by the Ministry of Health (MS). The intention was to generate changes in the model of care in force at the time, based on medical-curative actions, and its proposal was characterized by having the family as its nuclear unit of action, seeking integration with the community in which it is inserted and timely and early intervention. In addition, it was necessary to emphasize prevention and health education, which should then strengthen the principles of universality, integrality and equity advocated by the SUS (BRASIL, 1999a).

In 1996, the Ministry began to change the name from Program to Strategy, believing that it had the strategic potential to reorganize the health care model in Brazil (CORBO; MOROSINI, 2005). The Family Health Strategy (ESF) aims to reorganize primary care in Brazil, in line with the principles of the SUS, and is seen by the Ministry of Health and by state and municipal managers as a strategy for expanding, qualifying and consolidating primary care, because it favors a reorientation of the work process with greater potential to deepen the principles, guidelines and foundations of primary care, increase resolution and impact on the health situation of people and communities, as well as providing an important cost-effectiveness ratio (BRASIL, 2011a p. 17). 17).

Family Health is operationalized through the deployment of multi-professional teams in basic health units. These teams are responsible for monitoring a certain number of families in a given geographic area and work with "health promotion, prevention, recovery and rehabilitation of the most common diseases and conditions, as well as maintaining the health of this community" (BRASIL, 2011a).

An important point is the establishment of a multi-professional team (Family Health team) made up of at least: (I) a general practitioner, or specialist in Family Health, or Family and Community doctor; (II) a general nurse or specialist in Family Health; (III) a nursing assistant or technician; and (IV) community health agents. Oral health professionals can also be added to this composition: a general dental surgeon or specialist in Family Health, an oral health assistant and/or technician (BRASIL, 2011a).

It is still possible to implement the Community Health Agents Strategy in Basic Health Units, as a possibility for the initial reorganization of basic care, with a view to the gradual implementation of the ESF, or as a way of adding community agents to other ways of organizing basic care. Each Family Health team has been responsible for a maximum of 4,000 people, with the recommended average being 3,000 people, respecting equity criteria for this definition. It is recommended that the number of people per team should take into account the degree of vulnerability of the families in that territory, with the higher the degree of vulnerability, the fewer the number of people per team (BRASIL, 2011a).

In the municipality of Juiz de Fora, the ESF is in the process of being expanded and is facing challenges to solidify its position: defining the profile of the professionals who work in the PSF; specific training for professionals (specialization); continuing education for the teams; the inadequate infrastructure of the UAPS; the lack of rapport between team members (42% reported this difficulty); the differentiated remuneration among ESF professionals, causing discomfort in the teams; the majority of professionals not recording the activities carried out; the poor functioning of the referral and counter-referral system (SALDANHA, 2008). Saldanha (2008) reveals these challenges in his study and brings to light important elements for reflecting on and problematizing the ESF in the municipality. This research sought to evaluate the use of the health services network in Juiz de Fora, by means of surveys on users' opinions.

The study by Barra (2013) found that, in 2013, the municipality had 89 family health teams, representing 51.4% FHS coverage, serving a population of 265,197 people. The teams were located in 59 Primary Health Care Units (UAPS), distributed between urban and rural areas. In the urban area there were 32 Family Health Units (USF), two UAPS with the Community Health Agents Program (PACS) and ten traditional UAPS. In rural areas, there are five USFs, nine traditional UAPS and one mobile unit. Traditional health units are those staffed by general practitioners, obstetricians, gynecologists, pediatricians and nurses who do not work in teams.

The same study pointed out that the municipality has 76% PHC coverage, thus revealing the existence of 24% of totally uncovered areas, without an ESF and without a traditional unit, negatively impacting, in the author's assessment, the entire local health system, compromising the population's access (BARRA, 2013).

A recent study showed that primary care provides unspecific care for the elderly, which has a direct impact on their well-being. Therefore, there is an urgent need to develop social and welfare programs to meet the emerging needs of this population group. This portion of the population needs a view that is directed towards functionality and does not remain centered on the disease, given that, for them, health is not just about controlling and preventing aggravations of chronic non-communicable diseases, but in a process of interaction between physical and mental health, financial independence, functional capacity and social support (FERNANDES; SOARES, 2012).

3.3 HOME CARE

According to the Ministry of Health, Home Care in Primary Care/Family Health is a type of Home Care, inherent to the work process of the teams at this point of care. Its purpose is to respond to the health needs of a certain segment of the population with functional losses and dependence for carrying out activities of daily living (BRASIL, 2001 1b).

Considering the need to reformulate Ordinance No. 2.029/GM/MS, of August 24, 2011, which establishes Home Care within the scope of the Unified Health System (SUS) and, therefore, to readjust its rules and guidelines and to consolidate the Home Care modality, the Ministry of Health created Ordinance No. 2.527, on October 27, 2011, which redefined Home Care within the scope of the SUS. This ordinance states that Home Care (HC) consists of "an organizational and assistance device favorable to the implementation of new modes of care production and intervention at the various points of the Health Care Network (RAS), implying care centered on the user and their needs". According to this policy, HC began to integrate actions aimed at the individual at home, with the aim of humanizing care, de-hospitalization, minimizing the risk of hospital infection by reducing the length of hospitalization, when this becomes necessary (BRASIL, 2011b). Currently, Home Care is regulated by Ordinance 963 of May 27, 2013, which defines HC as:

A new type of health care, substitutive or complementary to existing ones, characterized by a set of health promotion, disease prevention and treatment and rehabilitation actions provided at home, with guaranteed continuity of care and integrated into health care networks (BRASIL, 2013 p.1).

According to Article 18 of this Ordinance, home care should be organized into three types: Type 1 Home Care (AD1), Type 2 Home Care (AD2) and Type 3 Home Care (AD3). In this paper, the emphasis will be on the AD1 modality, since it is the responsibility of primary care teams, through regular home visits at least once a month. Art. 20 characterizes AD1 as the type of care responsible for users who: have a controlled/compensated health problem and have difficulty or even the inability to travel to a health unit; those who need less complex care, including nutritional recovery, less frequently, with less need for health resources and within the service capacity of the Primary Health Care Units (UAPS); and do not fit the criteria for the AD2 and AD3 modalities, described in the same ordinance. The UAPS teams carrying out AD1 actions will be supported by the Family Health Support Centers (NASF)[1], as well as specialty and rehabilitation outpatient clinics. The equipment, permanent and consumable materials and the medical records of the users served in the AD1 modality will be kept in the physical structure of the UAPS themselves (BRASIL, 2013). It should be noted that the NASF has not been set up in the municipality where this research was carried out.

According to Brito *et al* (2013), home care is a health intervention strategy that enables practices that are closer to the concept of comprehensiveness, which, for Mattos (2004 cited by BRITO et al, 2013), has multiple meanings, one of which is horizontal comprehensiveness, in which it is proven that the answers to users' needs are often not achieved through a single contact with the health system, requiring sequential contacts with different services and monitoring of the therapeutic itinerary between them. The study by Brito *et al.* (2013) showed the vulnerability of Home Care within Primary Care, as it revealed important weaknesses with regard to the consolidation of the HV modality. The testimonies of the participants in this study related this fragility to the daily work of the ESF, which is marked by organizational and care conflicts that affect its work process and the performance of its activities.

In short, with regard to the Health of the Elderly, the legislation aimed at their care brings valuable contributions to this field, as it seeks to build policies aimed at comprehensive care, through the SUS, with special attention to the diseases that preferentially affect this age group, with an approach to prevention, promotion, protection and recovery of health. After

---

1 According to Decree 2488 of October 21, 2011, the **NASF** is an innovative strategy that aims to support, expand and improve health care and management in Primary Care/Family Health. Its requirements are, in addition to technical knowledge, responsibility for a certain number of Family Health teams and the development of skills related to the Family Health paradigm. They must also be committed to promoting changes in the attitude and performance of Family Health professionals and among their own team (NASF), including intersectoral and interdisciplinary action, health promotion, prevention, rehabilitation and healing, as well as humanizing services, continuing education, promoting comprehensiveness and the territorial organization of health services. The NASF should be made up of teams made up of professionals from different areas of knowledge, to work in support of and in partnership with the professionals of the Family Health teams, focusing on health practices in the territories under the responsibility of the Family Health team.

including the health of the elderly as one of the six priorities, the implementation of home care services became a guideline, with the aim of valuing the positive effect of the family environment on the elderly's health recovery process, as well as providing a beneficial effect for the health system, as a result of de-hospitalization. However, in practice, in a country where there are deficiencies in the public sector, particularly in the area of Public Health, as well as others such as Social Security, the elderly and their families remain on the margins of care, with punctual, incipient attention focused on the biomedical model of care, fragmenting the being, focusing on curing the disease and forgetting the being as a whole.

3.4 THE ELDERLY FAMILY CAREGIVER IN THE PROCESS OF CARING FOR OTHERS

Art can be seen primarily as a form of human-to-human contact in which feelings are transmitted. Therefore, caring can be seen as a form of artistic expression, an art, insofar as, from this practice, the human being becomes competent to openly express the individual feelings experienced and which, consequently, will be experienced by the recipient of the caring interaction. The art of caring emerges as a form of communication and the very expression of human feelings (WATSON, 2002). "The practice of caring is undoubtedly the oldest practice in the history of the world" (COLLIÈRE, 1999 p.25) and according to Boff (1999, p. 12.):

What opposes carelessness and neglect is care. Caring is more than an act; it is an attitude. Therefore, it encompasses more than a moment of attention, zeal and care. It represents an attitude of occupation, concern, responsibility and emotional involvement with others.

The act of caring implies respecting the person in all their peculiarities, from an individualized viewpoint, because each person is a unique being with their own particularities/lives and, only from this reflection, is decision-making promoted for their life and health project (WALDOW; BORGES, 2011).

Essentially, caring is an indispensable way of ensuring the continuity of human life, both individually and as a group, by pushing back death. In ancient times, caring included activities such as looking after the territory, chasing away the enemy, protecting the family and material goods, which were more closely linked to men. Women, in turn, took care of children, guaranteeing and preserving the continuity of human life (COLLIÈRE, 1989).

For Collière (1989), the essence of caring is the maintenance and continuity of life. The person carrying out the care becomes responsible for making up for the other person's temporary or permanent functional incapacity, and what we see is that, generally, this role falls to the family, since it is they, in the person of the family caregiver, who carry out and are responsible for the care. The responsibility of caring for dependent elderly people has been described by family caregivers as an exhausting and sometimes stressful task, due to the affective involvement and dependence, a process in which the caregiver prioritizes the physical and psychosocial well-being of the elderly person and thus restricts their own living (FERNANDES; GARCIA, 2009).

Nowadays, due to the overload of the health system, there is a tendency to reduce the length of stay of individuals hospitalized in health units as much as possible and to transfer a lot of care, which used to be considered hospital care, to Primary Health Care and Home Care services and, consequently, to families.

The changes that come with the aging process can bring numerous challenges, including the likelihood of developing chronic illness and/or disability. For many older people, this means assisting with the illness or disability of a loved one, such as a spouse, and then becoming a caregiver, which can also be a threat to the well-being of the caregiver (POULIN, et al., 2010).

The role of informal caregivers is therefore important in society, with significant implications for economic, social and human conditions. However, the caregiver becomes vulnerable to psychological disorders and may suffer burnout due to tension or overload, and may present symptoms such as: anxiety, depression and decreased self-esteem, stress, frustration, reduced social interaction, among others. These factors can trigger physical, psychological, emotional, social and financial problems, which therefore requires a targeted approach, with the aim of providing the necessary support and guidance to motivate both patient and caregiver. The aim is to achieve their active participation in therapy, with progress for the patient and improved quality of life for the family (CABRAL et al., 2014).

According to the Alliance for Aging Research (2011), 65.7 million caregivers make up 29% of the adult population in the United States and are found in 31% of all households. Of these, almost 49 million are caregivers of an elderly adult or patient, and between 20 and 25% of caregivers are aged 65 or over (ALLIANCE FOR AGING RESEARCH, 2011).

Elderly caregivers face a double risk: that of serving as a support by providing daily care to their loved one too often and suffering declines resulting from the aging process, which lead to the emergence of multiple chronic conditions and which have a direct impact on the well-being and health of the caregiver-care being cared for (MCGHAN et al., 2013).

According to Penrod *et al.* (2012), although the role of caregiver has been explored in various studies, there is still no recognition or way to support the needs of caregivers, especially from their perspective. There is a considerable body of literature on caregivers in general; however, studies of elderly caregivers and those who care for their spouses are limited by the use of cross-sectional designs (LAVELA; ATHER, 2010). Future research should carry out longitudinal studies over a longer follow-up period, as this will provide an understanding of the transition process and the challenges faced by elderly caregivers, as well as providing valuable information for this potentially vulnerable group of caregivers.

Family caregivers need and deserve support and appreciation from public policies and health professionals, especially with regard to the Family Health Strategy, which provides support for this population, especially since one of its members is the nurse, who can develop different types of care, especially help groups or networks that provide support for these caregivers (CELICH; BATISTELLA, 2007).

In order to offer quality care to caregivers and their families, it is necessary to know their life context, their culture and their belief systems. According to the authors, in their study, the caregivers pointed out that one form of self-care is faith. For them, faith is a form of self-care that helps them to have the strength and hope to continue on their way. Through faith in God, they are able to provide themselves with hope. In addition to their belief in a higher being, they reported that love and patience are essential for them to continue caring. Giving and dedication are related to sacrifice, which happens when people give themselves up in order to love others, without wanting anything in return (SEIMA; LENARDT; CALDAS, 2014).

In the multi-professional context of the ESF, the nurse's care process stands out, the planning of which is based on the health needs of the population (individuals, families and communities). In the context of health care for family caregivers, systematic assessment becomes an essential stage, with a view to exploring another dimension, which is spiritual care, in order to prevent and detect fatigue in these caregivers in advance. Nursing care must involve "helping the other person to take care of themselves by encouraging their existential potential to become" - this is "authentic care" (WALDOW, 1995 p.21/2).

The activity of caregiver has been culturally instituted in the care scenario for the elderly and, according to the Ministry of Health, in its publication *The Caregiver's Practical Guide*, this is defined as: "the person from the family or community who provides care to another person of any age, who is in need of care because they are bedridden, with physical or mental limitations, with or without remuneration" (BRASIL, 2008b).

Nurses work with the elderly in the field of health education, "care", based on knowledge of the diseases associated with the ageing process and the return of the elderly's functional capacity to carry out their activities, with the aim of meeting their basic needs and achieving their independence and well-being (DIOGO, 2007).

In addition, according to the author, nurses have the prospect of working in a multiplicity of services, from the community to the most technologically complex institutions. They are responsible for: education, care or direct assistance, advising, planning and coordinating services, teaching and evaluating the people who carry out these activities or those who are preparing to carry them out. Among the various fields in which nurses work in gerontology, we can mention communities, outpatient clinics, health centers and posts, homes, geriatric homes, nursing homes, centers or day hospitals, clinics and hospitals, among others. One of the aspects worth highlighting is teamwork, with the aim of providing comprehensive care for the elderly, i.e. to assist them in their bio-psychic and spiritual dimensions (DIOGO, 2007).

Studies carried out in Brazil and around the world show significant cultural characteristics, such as the fact that, in most cases, care is provided by a few or just one member of the family, called the main caregiver, who may or may not be a member of the family, and who carries out most of the care provided to the elderly in the home environment. It is also common for care to be carried out mainly by spouses and daughters, which gives women the role of "great caregivers", to whom this cultural and social role has been attributed, taking care of children, husbands and family members, but in many cases, this caregiver is also a frail person, already aging or in poor health (SARAIVA et al., 2007; SOUZA; CALDAS, 2008; VIEIRA et al., 2011; COUTO, 2013; MCGHAN et al., 2013).

A cross-sectional study aimed at identifying the correlates of caregiver burden among family caregivers of elderly Korean Americans found that female caregivers and spouses of the person being cared for were associated with greater burden. On the other hand, those with greater family support and greater management and self-care efficiency were associated with lower burden (CASADO; SACCO, 2012).

According to Araùjo; Paul; Martins (2009), who refer to the risk of alterations to the caregiver's health due to the wear and tear caused by the activities carried out daily in caring for dependent elderly people, the role of caregiver is arduous, a factor especially emphasized by elderly women who care for their elderly husbands. They show that they get so tired that they end up alienated from the world, but at the same time, they feel proud of the role they play (SILVA et al., 2014).

According to Seima; Lenardt and Caldas (2014), in a quantitative, cross-sectional and qualitative descriptive study carried out in Curitiba-PR, in a Reference Center for Alzheimer's Disease Care, caregivers reported that living with elderly people with chronic diseases, especially degenerative diseases, makes their routine stressful. Still for the authors, a decisive factor for greater wear and tear on caregivers is their advanced age. Caregivers over the age of 60, who carry out other activities associated with caregiving, live with the elderly person and care for them for a long time, are more likely to suffer from overload which, in general, leads them to be deprived of their social life, which is also a factor that can lead to increased overload.

The workload on the caregiver is sometimes significant. Therefore, it is of the utmost importance that there are other care options to be offered to families, in order to meet the needs of the elderly (BRASIL, 2008b). Most of the time, the responsibility taken on by the caregiver permeates a state of obligation, even when there is help from other family members, because the biggest commitment ends up being theirs. To overcome these difficulties, the caregiver uses the knowledge of the professional nurse, who will give them the security to deal with future circumstances in relation to caring for the patient, preparing the caregiver to practice simple care, which will facilitate and reduce the risks of worsening the clinical condition of the patient under their care. (MANOEL *et al.*, 2013).

This research adopts the concept of caregiver as the person who prioritizes the care needs of others (BRASIL, 2008b), the one who has the function of caring for someone with some degree of physical or mental dependence and who needs help (total or partial) to carry out the activities of daily living at home (MARCON *et al.*, 2006).

And with regard to the persistence in following a biomedical model centered on the disease, the person who provides the most assistance to the patient, "the caregiver", is left out of the picture, as this does not allow their work to be given the visibility it deserves and, even less, they have the support they need to carry out this role. Since the elderly family caregiver is the main person responsible for home care, this paper outlines their profile, exposes their feelings, difficulties, needs and recommends some actions that should be taken by the formal health system.

Therefore, it is the responsibility of public policies, services and health professionals to improve and develop actions that are truly family-centered, especially for the family caregiver, who is often elderly, taking into account their life context, beliefs and challenges, with a view to fostering the process of caring for others and for oneself, given that the caregiver often gives up their life in favor of assisting the person being cared for.

3.5 THE FAMILY AND THE HEALTH OF THE ELDERLY AT HOME.

Because it is a historically determined social institution that takes on different characteristics in a given socio-economic-political context, the family has undergone many changes. So many changes mean that we don't know exactly what a family is: we live with ideal models, while we see the progressive fragmentation of the nuclear model: mother, father and children (SZYMASNKI, 1992).

In the face of so many changes in what is known as the family, a change is emerging, called family ageing by Camarano *et al.* (2005), indicating that the number of families with at least one elderly person is growing every day. The changes in the constitution of families reflect a profound alteration in previously established values and in the functional roles played by one or more members (LOPES, 2007). The family structure can be nuclear or conjugal, which consists of a man, a woman and their children, whether biological or adopted, living in a shared family environment.

Nowadays, there has been a considerable emergence of a new family model, the so-called single-parent family. This is a variation on the traditional nuclear structure, due to social changes such as divorce, death, abandonment, illegitimacy or the adoption of children by a single person. We can also mention the extended or extended family, which consists of a broader structure, including the nuclear family plus direct or collateral relatives, with an extension of the relationship between parents and children to grandparents, parents and grandchildren (WHALEY AND WONG, 1989).

Thus, the family should be considered as a single social system, made up of a group of individuals, each with their own role to play and, although differentiated, they make up the functioning of the system as a whole. The most important thing when talking about any family structure is to consider that, necessarily, all of them will play a fundamental role in protecting the elderly. For this reason, it should be noted that the family is much more than an institution that biologically originates a being; it is, in particular, a web with distinct cultural and social characteristics (ATKINSON; MURRAY, 1989).

For Symanski (2002 p.9), the family is "an association of people who choose to live together for emotional reasons and assume a commitment to mutual care". However, the relevance of this does not come from the idealization of the family that still permeates the collective imagination, insofar as this space, while capable of producing "care, learning affections, building identities, bonds of belonging" (CARVALHO, 2003 p.15), can also generate a hostile environment, full of tyranny and inequalities.

However, for Elsen; Marconi e Silva (2004), the family is a health system, which includes a set of values, beliefs, knowledge and practices that guide family actions in promoting the health of its members, preventing and treating illness. And this system also includes a process of care, in which the family supervises the health condition of its members, makes decisions about the path to follow, constantly monitors and evaluates the health and illness of its members, asking for help from significant people and/or health professionals. For Sanches and Boemer (2002), the family is an essential part of the health of its members, since its basic function is to provide support, security and protection. The family acts affectionately, sometimes doing everything for its members; at other times it enables them to grow and mature so that they can follow their own paths (SANCHEZ; BOEMER, 2002).

Colliérè (1999) mentions that the family is the axis of care "(...) which in itself has a therapeutic value". As it is a living unit, it is in the family that the greatest number of informal caregivers are to be found, especially women, who have been doing this work since the dawn of humanity. However, for other authors, there are only four types of people in the world: those who have been cared for, those who are currently carers, those who will become carers and those who are dependent on a carer (MCSHERRY; JAMIESON, 2011).

At the extremes of life, whether in early childhood or in old age, there is a greater social limitation for the individual, who becomes dependent, sometimes vitally, on the society that surrounds and assists them. As the basis and root of the social structure is the family, it can be inferred that the study of the relationship between the elderly and their families is of primary importance in the study of the peculiarities of life and health at this stage (LEME, 2007).

Dealing with aspects involving ageing shows the visibility that the subject has been gaining. According to Lopes (2007), we are afraid of becoming old, because although the "good old age", explained by powerful and wise public figures, is increasingly publicized, the "denigrated old man" is part of our daily lives and is a frightening sight in our imagination.

According to Lopes and Calderoni (2002), the family is often unprepared to perceive and deal with the many transformations that occur with an ageing person and, even though they want to help, they are unable to position themselves appropriately. And when the family member takes on the role of caring for an elderly person, especially one affected by a chronic degenerative disease, they experience a cascade of changes to their family, social, financial and emotional routine (SEIMA; LENARDT; CALDAS, 2014).

Families, especially the main caregiver, are not prepared to deal with the new situation, further compromising the elderly person's clinical condition, as well as the family dynamic which is suddenly transformed by the presence of a dependent elderly person in the home. In these cases, the Family Health Strategy becomes an important ally because, as well as being part of mutual aid groups, it should contribute and help detect the necessary resources in the community to help improve the quality of care and life of the elderly person and their carer (NARDI; OLIVEIRA, 2008).

In maintaining the well-being of the elderly, the family has been identified by scholars as an important element, regardless of whether this assistance takes place in the activities of daily living or as emotional support (keeping company, helping to maintain or re-establish emotional ties, etc.). Thus, the family is a fundamental part of the concept of the elderly person, as part of the process of well-being, giving them autonomy, integration and acceptance in old age. Family vulnerability can lead to exclusion from social life, increasing the risk of pathologies and especially depression (CAMARANO, 2005).

Undoubtedly, elderly people want to continue to keep their homes, regardless of whether they are large or small, simple or totally comfortable, because it is in this environment, together with their belongings and memories, that they feel safe and self-confident (JARDIM, 2006).

The family certainly plays an important role in ensuring the well-being of their elderly relatives. The ideal would be for everyone to be able to remain with their family, but it has to be considered that the family, with all its socio-cultural and economic problems, is unlikely to be able to take care of its elderly dependents on its own. Faced with this situation, we refer to Article 229 of the 1988 Brazilian Constitution, which describes the duty and need for assistance between parents and children. "Parents have the duty to assist, raise and educate their minor children, and adult children have the duty to help and support their parents in old age, need or illness" (BRASIL, 1998). *In* article 230, we find the duty to support the elderly, whose responsibility should be shared between the family, society and the state (BRASIL, 1998).

For Cecilio (2011), health care management is the provision or availability of health technologies, according to the individual needs of each individual, at different times of their life, with a view to their well-being, safety and autonomy to continue with a productive and happy life. The management of care is based on five inseparable dimensions: individual, family, professional, organizational, systemic and societal, each of which offers specificities that should be known for reflection and intervention (CECILIO, 2011).

According to the author, the most central dimension is the individual dimension of health care management, i.e. each person can or has the potential to take care of themselves, while the family dimension of care management is one that acquires different values at different times in people's lives. This is a dimension of care management in which the privileged actors are family members, friends and neighbors. As a result of the accelerated ageing process of the Brazilian population, this dimension has taken on significant importance for health services and research. As a result, there are often conflicting relationships between caregivers and the cared-for, as a consequence of the complexity of family ties, the work overload for caregivers, the permanent demands for care, among others (CECILIO, 2011).

Health professionals are now looking at the family and not just the individual, as the family plays an important role in establishing and maintaining health. Therefore, for effective treatment to take place, the family will have to support care practices. The emergence of an illness within the family can lead to changes in life routines, causing suffering and anguish for family members and leading to an imbalance in the normal functioning of the people who live there, so involvement with the family is important for the patient's recovery (PENA; GONÇALVES, 2010).

In order to better meet the new demands, it is essential for health professionals to carefully and critically consider the peculiarities of their patient's family and try to adapt their health care to them. In this sense, it is of the utmost importance to know the context of life, the home, the environmental limitations, the routine of working hours, the dynamics of meals, etc. and the availability of support from family members, employees or relatives of the elderly person. (LEME, 2007)

This reflection on the complexity of today's family and the recognition of its importance in supporting old age aims to contribute to the training of professionals who will interfere in health policies, in order to collaborate in the difficult articulation of individual demands, family organization and institutional support (LOPES, 2006). When discussing the necessary conceptualization of the term "family" in the context of SUS care, it is defined as a collective subject, with particularities and experiences of internal conflicts, but with the potential to insert itself into the elaboration of a therapeutic plan for its dependent family member, considering its insertion in cultural contexts of intra- and extra-family care. Thus, outside the institutional confines of the health system, when investing in stimulating the development of personal skills for the self-care of a dependent family member, it must be recognized that the family shows a phenomenon of individualization, that is, each member of this family has a particular world that must be considered, as well as the peculiarities of each family (CASTRO, 2009).

3.6 SPIRITUALITY AND HEALTH

The study of spirituality in relation to health is essential, as research has shown that religiosity and spirituality are factors positively associated with psychological well-being, life satisfaction, happiness and improved physical and mental health. Religiosity gives meaning to people's lives and helps them deal with suffering and death (STROPPA and MOREiRA-ALMEiDA, 2008).

The subject of spirituality has been the object of many studies in the academic sphere, going beyond the boundaries of theology, thus determining other perspectives for a better understanding of this human phenomenon. Over the course of human history, it can be seen that spiritual and religious experiences differ according to the historical period, being directly influenced by the socio-historical and cultural context of the time (SOUZA, 2005; GUIMARAES, 2006).

Since the dawn of civilization, healing or medical practices have been intensely linked to spirituality. Even in modern times, when its consideration and appreciation have been outlawed from debate in research, professional practice and health care teaching environments, spirituality remains important in motivating and guiding many health professionals and patients (PENHA, 2008).

Seen through this mystical-religious lens, it was essentially carried out by shamans, priests, magicians and sorcerers, since illnesses were perceived as punishment sent by God or demonic possessions. Through Hippocrates, considered the "father of medicine", medical practices were absolved of religious mysticism, based on the basic foundations of propedeutics, as well as hygiene and nutrition measures as therapeutic practices. They believed that there was an immaterial nature in man, attached to the body, which instinctively regulated all the physiological functions of the organism and, if there was any imbalance, some pathological process would develop. They also considered other sources of energy, i.e. other higher immaterial entities (psyche, soul, etc.), which were linked to emotional aspects, intelligence and the human spiritual essence (TEIXEIRA, 2013).

From the 16th century onwards, with the advent of the Modern Age, scientific medicine began, with the Cartesian model predominating, for which the body and soul are independent. The emphasis was on studying the functioning of the human body, likening it to a machine, in other words, the human body should be studied in parts, just like a machine studied piece by piece. The modern world was rational and scientific, where positivism prevailed for understanding life (VASCONCELOS, 2006). During this period of scientific freedom, great advances were made in the field of experimental biology, with the emergence of academies, leading to an increase in physiology, pharmacology, anatomy, new discoveries about the causes of epidemics, and an appreciation of the concept of hygiene, among others (PENHA; SILVA, 2009).

Although some scholars have predicted that religiosity would tend to decrease drastically or even disappear, it is clear that this has not been the case, especially on the American continent, where there is a growing number of published works (MOREIRA-ALMEIDA;

LOTUFO NETO; KOENIG, 2008). According to Stroppa and Moreira-Almeida (2008), since the 1990s, a large number of articles have been published in academic literature in the areas of health and the relationship between religion and health. National and international researchers have dedicated themselves to studies on the subject by developing valid and reliable tools to access it (PANZINE; ROCHA; BANDEIRA; FLECK, 2007).

Elucidating the definition of the term "spirituality" is no simple task, as it might seem, because in the West the word has a great deal of tradition attached to it, i.e. it is entangled with the meaning of religiosity. According to King and Crowther (2004), there is a tendency to use these expressions synonymously, giving them similar meanings. However, spirituality can be conceptualized in different ways and from different points of view, since it is a field of study in formation and has attracted an increasing number of interested parties (VASCONCELOS, 2006). A number of studies have shown that nurses, doctors, philosophers, psychologists and sociologists look at spirituality and religion from different perspectives, bringing together various possible facets of the approach, as shown below:

The results of a study by Dyson and Cobb (1997) showed that spirituality was strongly associated with the concept of religiosity, above all due to the fact that, when they carried out the study, there was little research on this specific subject. Those that did exist sought to establish a relationship between religious influence and the health-disease process. On the other hand, in this study, spirituality was also related to a good relationship with God, with others and with oneself, in order to achieve meaning in life (DYSON; COBB 1997).

For Allport (1950), religious experience was something fundamentally personal, subject to the laws of psychological evolution. For the author, religion was a very important factor in the integration of the personality, claiming that it was man's effort to unite with creation and the Creator, with the aim of expanding and completing his own personality. According to the author, religion has been described in terms of two fundamental aspects that permeate religious experience: intrinsic religiosity and extrinsic religiosity. Extrinsic religiosity, or less spiritualized religiosity, is found among those who "inherit" their religious beliefs. There is no reflexive tendency when choosing a religious entity or philosophy and, in this case, divinity tends to be an instrument for satisfying impulsive or egocentric desires. In the intrinsic or more spiritualized practice, a form of religiosity associated with the search for meaning, unity and transcendence and a search for the maximum of human potential, there is a search to overcome comfort and social convention, seeking meaning and an increased commitment to the belief or religion (ALLPORT, 1950).

For GEERTZ (1978), religious experience was understood as individual, that is, different for each individual, even if they shared the same belief. For Lotufo Neto (1997), spirituality is the individual's quest to achieve a full, meaningful life, oriented towards something greater, non-material, that lies beyond, through which one discovers some form of dependence or recognition of this higher being. Spirituality would comprise the "personal process aimed at relating oneself to the essential higher power". According to the author, "God is a living, personal and invisible spirit, the creator of life and the perfect model to be sought after" (LOTUFO NETO, 1997). In this way, religion is "the oldest and most enduring human institution", and therefore inconceivable to separate from the cultural history of humanity. The justification for such a long duration is due to the fact that religion must play a relevant role for the individual and society (LOTUFO NETO, 1997).

Religious experience is unique, different from everyday experiences, it affects core perceptions about yourself and life, it can change notions about who you are and the meaning or significance of your life. Religious experience is complex from a psychological point of view, involving emotions, beliefs, attitudes, values, behaviors and social environment. It transcends these psychological categories and gives the individual a sense of wholeness (LOTUFO NETO; 1997, p. 3).

Spirituality can be defined as something that brings meaning and purpose to people's lives and also functions as a factor that contributes to people's health and quality of life. This definition is found in all cultures and societies and is expressed as an individual search, through participation in religious groups that have something in common, such as faith in God, naturalism, humanism, family and art (PUCHALSKI, 1999).

The spiritual basis comes from an emblematic and fascinating reality that takes hold of the human being and manifests the presence of something sublime, at the same time in such a simple way that it creates possibilities to be lived in everyday life. For Boff (2001), spirituality is the ability to experience an inner strength capable of surpassing one's own abilities; it is the art of allowing oneself to be invaded and guided in life by the experience of transcendence. According to the author, spirituality is the dive we make into ourselves. From the moment we return to our inner selves, sometimes through meditation techniques, we plunge into the depths of our being and, by experiencing reality as a whole, we are experiencing our spirituality (BOFF, 2001).

In her study, Tanyi (2002) identified that spirituality has been understood in a controversial way, sometimes treated as synonymous with religiosity, sometimes associated with the demands of religious beliefs, and sometimes radically unrelated. Rare were the findings of a good relationship between the two terms.

For Hufford (2005), spirituality refers to the realm of the spirit (God or gods, souls, angels, demons), something extra-physical, what was once called the supernatural. Spirituality is a personal relationship with the transcendent, in a more general sense it includes religion and is an aspect of the core of religion. It represents the existence of individuals who are "spiritual" but not religious, or even individuals who are totally skeptical and notably not spiritual. For the same author, religion is an institutionalized form of spirituality. Religions are institutions organized around the concept of spirit (HUFFORD, 2005).

For Dalgalarrondo (2008), religiosity and spirituality can be understood as broad dimensions that are independent of institutionalized designations of religion. Religiosity and spirituality are experienced in different ways during human development, in other words, religiosity undergoes transformations throughout the life cycle.

While many authors adhere to the idea that religion can be a form of spirituality, others, like those mentioned above, believe that spirituality always has to do with the transcendent. On the other hand, some authors consider the possibility of a spirituality of an immanent nature, in other words, nothing beyond the physical body, neither God nor spirit. According to the materialist philosopher Comte-Sponville (2007), who defends the broad idea of spirituality, the spirit is not a substance but a function of the brain, through which the individual is in control. This philosopher points out that

All religion belongs, at least in part, to spirituality; but not all spirituality is necessarily religious. Whether or not you believe in God, the supernatural or the sacred, in any case you will find yourself confronted with the infinite, eternity, the absolute - and with yourself. Nature is enough for that. Truth is enough for that. Our own transient and relative finitude is enough. We could not otherwise think of ourselves as relative, nor as ephemeral, nor as finite. (COMTE-SPONVILLE, 2007:129)

For Giovanetti (2005), spirituality is an activity of our spirit and doesn't necessarily imply faith in some transcendent being, which is a necessary characteristic for experiencing religiosity. Boff (2001) says that spirituality has to do with experience and not with dogmas, rites or celebrations. The word "spirituality" indicates any experience that can produce profound transformation within each person and that leads to personal integration and integration with other people.

In the 19th century, Florence Nightingale described spirituality from a phenomenological-existentialist perspective, which brings strongly conscious knowledge in relation to the divine presence. According to Macrea (2001) and reported by Penha (2008):

We can't call the love, admiration, reverence or trust that one human being has for another human being. These we call humanizing influences; but feelings arising from the awareness of a presence of a nature greater than the human, disconnected from what is material; this we can call a spiritual influence; and being aware is the highest ability of our nature (PENHA, 2008).

In this paper, we will adopt the definition of spirituality/religiosity according to Koenig; Mcculloug and Larson (2001), who explain spirituality as a personal search for answers to essential questions about life and its meaning, as well as relationships with the sacred and the transcendent, which may or may not lead to the development of religious rituals and the formation of a community. Religiosity is the extent to which an individual believes in, follows and practices a religion. It can be organizational (attending church or a religious temple) or non-organizational (praying, reading books, watching religious programs on television). And religion is an organized system of beliefs, practices, rituals and symbols, designed to facilitate proximity to the sacred or transcendent (God, higher power or supreme truth/reality) and promote understanding of relationships and responsibility for others living in the same community (KOENIG; MCCULLOUG; LARSON, 2001; MOREIRA-ALMEIDA; LOTUFO NETO; KOENIG, 2006; KOENIG; KING; CARSON, 2012).

After different perspectives, alternatives can be found in the search for a new way of thinking about health work, focused on humanization, health care and care for the individual or social groups, in an integrated view of the human being, as a plural being endowed with reason, emotion, intuition, sensitivity and spirituality, which must be understood in its multiple approaches, leaving aside a fragmented view of symptomatology or medicalization. All of this is done through a posture of understanding, acceptance and dialogue in search of solutions to improve the quality of life of the less-favored working classes (GUIMARÂES, 2006).

According to Vasconcelos (2006), the development of sensitivity, the use of reason combined with emotional aspects and intuition becomes essential for quality care, with a humanistic and therefore integrated view of the human being. It must therefore be understood in its multiple aspects, disregarding fragmentation and the process of medicalization of the being. And this is possible through spirituality. However, for the author, despite the fact that spirituality is linked to the area of health, both from the perspective of the professional and the individual to be cared for, it is commonly hidden among professionals, in general, due to the difficulty of discussing it (VASCONCELOS, 2006). According to Lucchetti *et al.* (2012), this difficulty stems from the fact that professionals, especially in the medical field, are not trained to deal with patients' spiritual beliefs and that many barriers are created by them, such as lack of time and knowledge, which are used as excuses for not paying attention to the spiritual dimension of the patient/user.

In a study carried out in the United Kingdom, the preliminary results of a descriptive survey showed that nurses recognize spirituality as a fundamental aspect of nursing care and that meeting patients' spiritual needs improves the quality of care in general. The data also shows that there was some uncertainty about the boundary between personal belief and professional practice. However, despite this recognition of the attention given to the spiritual dimension, the professionals interviewed advocate the formal integration of spirituality into nursing training programs, the need for professional training and the support of social agencies, so that they can meet the spiritual needs of their patients effectively (MCSHERRY; JAMIESON, 2011, 2013).

According to Penha and Silva (2012), religiosity and spirituality have become a watershed for the new era, especially as it has been shown that religious/spiritual beliefs and practices have had a major impact on helping people cope with the most diverse circumstances of imbalance in their health, as well as preparing them for death, and even on professionals' interpersonal relationships.

Although less common, spiritual or religious beliefs can negatively interfere with health treatment, leading to health problems or worsening the outcome of a disease. It is important for health professionals to be aware of when spiritual or religious beliefs may worsen health or conflict with appropriate treatment. Religion can be responsible for personal judgments, it can become rigid, inflexible, restrictive and limiting; but it can also encourage magical thinking, as people pray hoping for a cure, as if God had to fulfill every human wish. If the physical cure doesn't come promptly, the individual tends to feel resentful, saying that the prayer wasn't answered and that God doesn't care, or, worse still, that the illness was sent as revenge from God, as a form of punishment for their sins. Another worrying form is when religion is used in place of prescribed medical treatment. Treatments are avoided or even discontinued on religious grounds. Patients may stop taking their medication after attending a healing service to "demonstrate their faith", potentially having a negative impact on their illness and their response to medical treatment (KOENIG. 2005; LUCCHETTI et al., 2010).

Based on the various definitions of spirituality and religion, it is understood that there is no consensus among researchers as to the meaning of religiosity and spirituality. They are considered to be culturally relevant factors and cannot therefore be reduced to a simple phenomenon, as they are multidimensional and complex constructs at various levels, such as: the biological, the affective, the cognitive, the moral, the relational, the level of personality and self-identity. A growing body of research shows that religiosity and spirituality can be positively associated with health and well-being. However, there is also a negative side, both in terms of mental health and emotional suffering.

There is a growing body of evidence on the relationship between religiosity/spirituality and physical and mental health, which indicates that this is a promising field of research. Finally, it is essential that, in the course of this challenging task, we spontaneously set out, regardless of whether we have materialistic or spiritual beliefs or not, whether we are convinced or not, whether we have religious attitudes or not, because what we really need to do is, consciously explore this abstract relationship that exists between the phenomenon of spirituality and health, so that we can improve and deepen our knowledge and concept of the human being, in a broad and comprehensive way, as well as reconducting new therapeutic approaches.

3.6.1 Spirituality of the elderly

Snodgrass and Sorajjakool (2011) aimed to explore the relationship between spirituality and ageing, with a focus on the factors that can result in an increase in spirituality among the elderly. They found that the aging process and the acquisition of knowledge, through the difficulties suffered over the course of life, significantly influence the opportunity to embrace human finitude, to recognize the continuity of life and to grow in clarity about God (SNODGRASS; SORAJJAKOOL, 2011).

Carl Gustav Jung's thinking emphasizes the importance of studying man's spiritual dimension, with an emphasis on the ageing phase, because as we get older, in difficult times, crises and illnesses, coping based on the spiritual dimension has been proven to be vitally important and meaningful. The ageing process seems to generate a need to look back on life and, from there, a new balance emerges in the face of the changes related to growing old (MONTEIRO, 2006).

According to the model of personality development proposed by Erik Erikson (1998), which presents a holistic and dynamic view of life, there is a pressing need to constantly re-elaborate and re-signify life throughout the life cycle, which allows the individual to review behaviors and deliberate on old crises as they age. In its initial approach, the study describes eight stages of human development, stating that each phase of development presents its own challenges, which the author calls crises. However, the person who has overcome the previous crises and is inserted in a psychosocial context that helps them overcome the current difficulties will not allow hopelessness to take over their life (ERIKSON, 1998).

After the loss of her husband, Joan Erikson developed the ninth stage of human development. According to the author, around the age of 80 or more, when physical health begins to deteriorate progressively, there are losses of friends and family members, and death itself becomes a closer reality. If the elderly person manages to overcome the dystonic elements of the experiences of the ninth stage, they will probably follow the path that leads to Gerotranscendence (ERIKSON, 1998).

According to Tornstam (1997), human development towards Gerotranscendence takes place on three levels, the first of which is called cosmic: an increased sense of unity with the universe, when the individual seeks to redefine the perception of time, space, life and death. There is an increasing affinity with past and future generations. On the second level, the redefinition of the *self* involves a decrease in egocentrism and a decline in material interest, and these characteristics of the ego often combine with the characteristics on the third social level, which is characterized by a decline in superfluous social contacts and an increase in the time devoted to meditation (TORNSTAM, 1997). For Braam *et al.* (2006), Gerotranscendence has been conceptualized as a potential development that accompanies normal ageing. The theory of Gerotranscendence consists of a concept that explains the aging process by idealizing a special state of mind, when there is a shift in perspective from a materialistic and pragmatic view of the world to a more cosmic and transcendent view of aging (TORNSTAM, 1989; GAMLIEL, 2001).

The study by Braam *et al.* (2006) found a significant positive association between cosmic transcendence and meaning in life for the elderly. This association was more pronounced among participants with less religious involvement, especially in the case of women over 75 and widows. The study suggests that the personal relevance of cosmic transcendence depends on cultural factors as well as the individual life context.

According to Monod *et al.* (2010), spirituality is considered an essential component of a multidimensional approach to be used in geriatric care for elderly patients with health problems. Spirituality has also been identified as a positive way of coping with illness, disability or life-threatening conditions. According to the authors, several studies have documented significant associations between spirituality and better health: mental, physical and functional (MONOD, 2010).

In Brazil, the study by Lucchetti *et al.* (2011), with the aim of evaluating the relationship between religiosity and mental health in situations of hospitalization, pain, disability and quality of life of elderly people in an outpatient rehabilitation setting, concluded that religiosity is significantly related to fewer depressive symptoms, improved quality of life and a reduction in cognitive impairment. Religious involvement can play a protective role in the body, prevent health problems, help with recovery or adaptation to problems and can be considered a factor in coping with chronic conditions and the disability they cause (LUCCHETTI *et al.*, 2011).

In her study, Freitas (2014) mentions the positive effects of religiosity and spirituality on health and well-being, in people's perceptions, especially in critical or stressful situations, including aging and improving the mental health of depressed elderly people, in the perspective of the end of life, among others. The author also discusses the variety of ways in which religious involvement positively influences the lives and health of individuals, acting as social support in coping with life's diversities (FREITAS, 2014).

However, although studies are advancing every day on the subject in question, there is still a gap between theory and practice. And even when professionals recognize the importance of religiosity and spirituality in the health/disease process, they don't know how to combine medical knowledge with culture, common sense and other knowledge production in patient care, especially when it comes to managing the relationship between religiosity and physical or mental health. In general, professionals often feel unprepared and insecure to deal with their patients' religious issues, as they claim they lack the training to deal with the subject properly (FREITAS, 2014).

4. METHODOLOGICAL PATH

But the parts of the world all have such relationships and such a connection with each other that I find it impossible to understand one without reaching the others, and without penetrating the whole.

PASCAL

4.1 TYPE OF STUDY AND THEORETICAL-METHODOLOGICAL APPROACH

In order to understand the issue and achieve the proposed objectives, we decided to carry out a qualitative study to understand the process of caring for others by elderly family caregivers from different socio-economic and cultural backgrounds.

According to Polit, Beck and Hungler (2004), qualitative research methods deal with the complex aspects inherent in human beings, their ability to shape and create their own experiences, as well as the idea that truth is the possibility of arriving at a cluster of realities. Consequently, qualitative research emphasizes understanding the human experience as it is lived and reported by the subjects taking part in the research. Qualitative methodology applied to health not only seeks to study the phenomenon itself, but to understand its meaning in the individual or collective sphere (TURATO, 2005).

Qualitative research is multi-methodological in focus, encompassing an interpretive and naturalistic approach to its subject. This means that qualitative researchers investigate facts in their natural *setting*, seeking to make sense of or interpret phenomena in terms of the meanings that people bring to them (DENZIN; LINCOLN, 1994). There are a variety of ways to carry out qualitative research and, in this study, we opted for the *Grounded* Theory method.

4.1.1 Grounded Theory

This research used Data-Driven Theory (DDT), devised by American sociologists Barney Glaser and Anselm Strauss, who called it *"Grounded Theory"*. Both were sociology professors at the University of California and pooled their knowledge and experience to develop techniques for analyzing qualitative data. This approach derives from Symbolic Interactionism, which, according to Blumer (1986), is a theoretical perspective centered on the interaction between people, apprehending, when interacting, the action, perception, interpretation and reaction of things in relation to the other. It also allows data to be collected in natural settings, where data collection, analysis and theory are closely related (STRAUSS; CORBIN, 2008). According to Charmaz (2009, p. 24), PDT "serves as a way of learning about the worlds we study and as a method for developing theories to understand them".

Symbolic interactionism seeks to reveal the meaning that the world has for each individual, as well as the kind of influence it exerts on their attitudes and decision-making. From this theoretical perspective, human groups or societies are seen as a set of human beings who are in action, through the multiple activities that individuals carry out in their lives, how they relate to each other and how they deal with these situations (BLUMER, 1969).

The purpose of PDT is to understand social phenomena in the context in which they occur, observing the interrelationship between meaning and action and, from there, developing a theoretical model (STRAUSS, CORBIN, 2008). From the 1960s onwards, PDT, which until then had been widely used in education, began to influence the development of nursing knowledge. The main focus of the theory's contribution to transversal nursing knowledge was on adaptation to illness, infertility, adaptation and nursing interventions, as well as the study of vulnerable people and groups (STREUBERT and CARPENTER, 1999), as in the case of this study, in which we are working with elderly caregivers who look after another elderly person at home, whose health is compromised, who has one or more chronic illnesses and therefore needs specific nursing care at home, just as much as the person being cared for.

PDT is an important research method for the study of phenomena in the field of nursing. The method explores the richness and diversity of human experience and contributes to the development of middle-range theories in nursing, as well as helping to theoretically explain gaps between theory, research and practice (STREUBERT; CARPENTER, 1999).

Strauss and Corbin define methodology as a way of thinking about social reality and studying it, while method is characterized by "the set of procedures and techniques for collecting and analyzing data" (STRAUSS and CORBIN, 2002, p. 3). They also highlight three main elements in qualitative research: firstly, the data that emanates from various sources, such as interviews, observations, documents, records, films and photographs. Secondly, the methods used to interpret and organize the data, which include: conceptualizing and reducing the data; developing categories according to their properties and dimensions and; rationalizing through propositions. These procedures are known as codification. The analytical process also includes non-statistical sampling, memos and diagrams. Finally, the third refers to the publication and public presentation of the results.

Grounded theory is an inductive methodology that approaches the subject under investigation without a preconceived theory. Used in the development of a thesis based on systematically collected and analyzed data, the theory emerges during the course of the research and is based on the continuous interaction between analysis and data collection (STRAUSS & CORBIN, 2008).

From this perspective, theory is what the researcher ends his work with and not how he begins it. It is not what is going to be tested, but what is concluded after research and the comparative analysis of the resulting data. Unlike formal theories, which provide the concepts and hypotheses needed to explain the phenomenon, in TFD, the researcher builds a theory from the specific observation of the phenomenon and not by applying a pre-established theory to explain it (DICK, 2005). Thus, because it is a general method of constant comparative analysis, the PDT is often referred to as a comparative method (GASQUE, 2007).

One of the advantages discussed by Fragoso, Recuero and Amaral (2011) is the fact that PDT values the researcher's contact with the object and encourages the creation of a sensitivity to the data. Experiencing the empirical field also allows the researcher to observe new elements and build their perceptions by systematically analyzing and reflecting on the data found in the field.

According to Fragoso, Recuero and Amaral (2011), although it is not a simple method, PDT is extremely interesting because it proposes analysis concomitantly with the data collection process, thus allowing theory to emerge from the empirical. The purpose of TFD, then, is to establish a reliable theory that can shed light on a particular area of study. To this end, some of the method's criteria must be followed with methodological rigor: data collection; coding/categorization; and writing the theory.

According to Strauss and Corbin (2008), there is a case for alternating data collection and analysis. As well as allowing validation based on emerging concepts, it also allows concepts and hypotheses to be validated as they are developed. Those considered to be "unadjustable" can then be rejected or modified during the research process.

For Gasque (2007), when using this methodology, the researcher first needs to leave their knowledge in a "state of suspension" so that the theory can emerge, in other words, they must be open to the new and the unexpected.

According to Levacov (2003), an important piece of information that should be noted is that the theory to be created does not only arise to explain a phenomenon, but also provides a reference scheme for action. Therefore, the TFD aims to clarify a phenomenon present in reality and this process will take place through qualitative analysis, which can bring new knowledge to the area of the phenomenon (STRAUSS; CORBIN, 2008).

Although basing concepts on data is the main characteristic of TFD, the creativity of researchers is also essential. Thus, with qualitative data, the researcher must be able to base their considerations on critical and creative thinking, both in science and in the art of analysis. Several techniques are used to collect data in the TFD, including: interviews, observation, memos, speeches, letters, biographies, autobiographies, library research, among others

(DICK, 2005).

The research process in PDT takes place in five stages: the collection of empirical data; open coding; axial coding; selective coding; and the construction of the research report (STREUBERT; CARPENTER, 1999; STRAUSS; CORBIN, 2008). Fundamentally, then, a concise description of the tool is necessary before starting to collect data, because "approaching the field is one of the crucial moments of the PDT" (FRAGOSO, RECUERO and AMARAL, 2011, p. 89).

Regarding coding or analysis, Strauss and Corbin (2008, p. 25) indicate that analysis is the interaction between researchers and data, and is the result of the encounter between science and art. It is science in that it characterizes and maintains the rigour required of it and bases analysis on data. In line with this, art manifests itself through creativity, in the researchers' ability to name categories, ask stimulating questions, make comparisons and extract an innovative, integrated scheme, as well as allowing tone to emerge from the mass of raw data. Given the data collected, TFD procedures are followed to help ensure rigor in the creation process. These procedures, however, are not designed to be followed dogmatically, but rather to be used creatively and flexibly. They are called coding, which in turn is an integral part of the theory-building process and requires a great deal of concentration at the risk of losing the essence of the testimonies. This process aims to give methodological rigor to the process of preparing the data for analysis (STRAUSS and CORBIN, 2008). Strauss and Corbin (2008, p. 26) describe the coding process as follows:

1)   Building instead of testing theory.

2)   Provide researchers with the analytical tools to deal with masses of raw data.

3)   To help analysts consider alternative meanings for phenomena.

4)   Being systematic and creative at the same time.

5)   Identify, develop and relate the concepts that are the building blocks of theory (STRAUSS and CORBIN, 2008, p. 26).

The first stage, represented by data collection, can be done through formal or semi-structured interviews, informal interviews, observation, journals, documents or a combination of these sources. The collection of relevant data provides solid material for the construction of a meaningful analysis. The data reveals the opinions, feelings, intentions and actions of the participants, as well as the contexts of their lives. Obtaining this data involves dense description, such as writing up observations from field notes, personal accounts from participants in writing and/or compiling detailed narratives (such as transcribing recorded interviews) (CHARMAZ, 2009).

The interview process can adopt a dialogical line between interviewee and interviewer. The researcher develops some questions for the fieldwork and, as soon as the data begins to emerge, they are discarded (STRAUSS; CORBIN, 2008). As answers emerge, different questions may arise and, in this case, it should be emphasized that the generating question technique can be used, i.e. the one that allows for a more flexible and comprehensive display of the topic in question (SANTOS, 2009). The instrument can also be restructured by changing the focus of the questions, with the aim of explaining and discovering the reality being investigated, or in the way it is questioned, with the aim of getting closer to the subjects' understanding and thus extracting as much information as possible (DE CARVALHO DANTAS et al., 2009).

Observation is a qualitative research technique that examines an event within a context with all the senses and is used to describe a previously defined problem. It requires training so that the senses can be focused on the object of research, by observing the subject's non-verbal behavior, i.e. observation can be a valuable collection resource, since it makes it possible to understand what cannot be expressed, or what the subject cannot express in words (STRAUSS; CORBIN, 2008). Observation is important for understanding what cannot be said or written, such as the environment, behavior and non-verbal language, with the aim of knowing and understanding reality. It requires memory training, and it is essential to take short notes in a field diary, which must be expanded later (ViCTORA; KNAUTH; HASSEN, 2000). Therefore, it is necessary to record it in a field diary, which is a place where the researcher takes notes, such as their impressions of conversations and observations of behavior (MINAYO, 2010).

The second stage, open coding, is based on the analytical process, through which concepts are identified and their properties and dimensions discovered in the data. In this stage, the concepts are revealed, named and developed; the researcher must open up the text and expose the thoughts, ideas and meanings it contains. Without this first analytical step, the other stages of analysis and the communication that follows may not take place properly (STRAUSS; CORBIN, 2008). This stage can be carried out in different ways, including line-by-line analysis, which was adopted in this study, and involves a thorough examination of the data, sentence by sentence and sometimes word by word, always aiming to capture the subjects' point of view on the phenomenon being researched. This is the most time-consuming method, but produces the best results (STRAUSS; CORBIN, 2008).

The third stage, axial coding, is the process of relating categories to their subcategories. It has this name because this coding takes place around the axis of a category, associating categories at the level of properties and dimensions. The aim of this coding is to begin the process of regrouping the data that was divided during open coding. The categories are related to their subcategories in order to generate more precise and complete explanations of the phenomena. Although axial coding has a different objective to open coding, these steps are not necessarily sequential analytical steps. It requires the analyst to have some categories, but a sense of how the categories are related always begins to emerge during open coding (STRAUSS; CORBIN, 2008).

In this phase, the aim is to discover the main problem in the social scene described by the subjects participating in the study and how they express the problem. It is important to note that coding helps the researcher to integrate the categories and the aim is to gather the data, making connections between the categories and subcategories, taking into account the data collected, considering the so-called paradigm, in order to delve deeper into the theory that emerges (STRAUSS; CORBIN, 2008).

The fourth stage is selective coding, the process of integrating and refining the theory. In integration, the categories are organized around a central explanatory concept, the central category (or basic category), which represents the main theme of the research. Integration takes place over time, beginning with the first steps of the analysis and usually not ending until the final draft. Once a commitment to the central idea has been achieved, the main categories are related to it through explanatory statements of relationships. Various techniques can be used to facilitate the integration process, including: speaking or writing the storyline, using diagrams, classifying and reviewing memos (STRAUSS; CORBIN, 2008).

This phase stands out as the moment when the categories are refined. This process seeks to integrate the categories and subcategories until the central category is defined, which should be present in most of the reports. The central category represents the main theme of the research, which gives cohesion to the Theory, generating the causal conditions, the context, the intervening conditions, the strategies and the consequences, theoretical relationships through which the categories are related to each other and to the central category (STRAUSS and CORBIN, 2008).

As criteria for choosing the central category, Strauss and Corbin (2008) suggest that it should have analytical power. What gives it this power is its ability to bring together the other categories to form an explanatory framework. Strauss (1987, p. 36) provides a list of criteria that can be applied to a category to define whether it qualifies as central:

1.   It must be central, meaning that all other important categories can be linked to it;

2.   They should often appear in the data, i.e. in all or almost all cases, there are indicators pointing to this concept;

3.   The explanation that results from the relationship between the categories is logical and consistent;

4.   The name or phrase used to describe the core category should be sufficiently abstract so that it can be used to do research in other substantive areas, leading to the development of a more general theory;

5.   As the concept is refined analytically through integration with other concepts, the theory gains depth and greater explanatory power;

6.   The concept can explain variations and also the main point of the data (STRAUSS, 1987, p. 36).

Finally, there is the fifth stage, which corresponds to the production of the research report and should give readers an idea of the sources of the data, how they were interpreted and how the concepts were integrated (STREUBERT; CARPENTER, 1999).

In PDT, the researcher finds himself in a naturalistic setting, where it is not possible to control his presence or try to withdraw from the study. In this case, they bring their personal experience to the study, emphasizing their understanding of the problem (STREUBERT; CARPENTER, 1999). The research question in this approach identifies the phenomenon to be studied and sampling is determined by the generation of data and its analysis. Researchers who use the TFD continue to collect data until saturation occurs, which, in the case of this theory, is considered to be when the data analyzed no longer allows for the creation of new codes or the expansion of existing ones (STREUBERT; CARPENTER, 1999). Therefore,

A category is considered saturated when no new information seems to emerge during coding, i.e. when no new properties, dimensions, conditions, actions/interactions or consequences are seen in the data (STRAUSS &CORBIN, 2008, p.135).

Therefore, based on the above, this methodology was chosen in order to gain a deeper understanding of the daily life of the elderly caregiver, with a view to the process of caring for another elderly person at home.

4.2 ACTION STRATEGIES

4.2.1 Research scenario

The research was carried out in the Minas Gerais municipality of Juiz de Fora, whose estimated population in 2014, according to the IBGE, was 550,710 inhabitants (IBGE, 2014).

The municipality is a hub of the southeastern macro-region of Minas Gerais, a reference in health for 94 municipalities (JUIZ DE FORA, 2014a), due to the existence of highly complex outpatient and hospital health services, distributed between public and private providers, for-profit or not-for-profit, for the most part (FARAH, 2006; ALBERTONI, 2014).

According to the 2014 Basic Sanitation Plan, the municipality of Juiz de Fora has an excellent treated water supply service,

and, in 2010, the coverage of the services provided was almost 100%, which is positive for the population's quality of life (JUIZ DE FORA, 2014b).

Currently, 63 UAPS are part of the network of services offered in Primary Health Care (PHC) in the municipality of Juiz de Fora (JUIZ DE FORA, 2014c). According to the SUS health care organization model, the initial setting in which subjects are identified in the health services network is Primary Health Care, represented by Primary Health Care Units. The study included elderly caregivers living in the areas covered by the UAPS, located in the north of the municipality. This region was chosen because it has an extensive urban area and is far from the city center, where the main institutions for the care and attention to the health of the elderly are located.

The health structure of the municipality of Juiz de Fora is divided into well-defined health regions, with the aim of strengthening PHC and its interfaces with the various units at other levels of care. The north/northwest and north zones are called regions seven and eight, respectively, and include the following neighborhoods: Region 7 (north and northwest) - Esplanada, Monte Castelo, Industrial, Jardim Natal, Milho Branco, Jóquei Clube I, Jóquei Clube II and Cidade do Sol; Region 8 (north) - Nova Era, Sao Judas Tadeu, Santa Cruz, Benfica, Vila Esperança and Barreira do Triunfo. According to the 2014-2017 Municipal Health Plan, the region has 117,238 inhabitants and 14 Primary Health Care Units, three of which operate as a traditional unit and the others as an ESF, totaling 30 health teams, which supported the choice for the research (JUIZ DE FORA, 2014d).

In order to carry out this research, authorization was requested and obtained from the Municipal Health Department and the Nursing School Management, as shown in Appendices A and B.

4.2.2 Research participants

The TFD is a circular method and therefore allowed the researcher to change the focus of attention and look for other directions, according to the data that emerged on the scene. It also allowed her to return to the field as many times as necessary, so that a theoretical construct could emerge from the data. This study was saturated with seven participants; however, in order to compare the data so as to allow a reliable interpretation of the testimonies and to obtain the scientific rigor that is required of a study of this nature, we returned to the field for three more interviews, following the guidelines of the reference. The eighth, ninth and tenth interviews were focused on direct questions about the phenomenon in question; however, it is important to point out that the direction was given only after the interviewee had said something about his values and beliefs, with the sole aim of not influencing his answers, based on methodological rigor.

For this study, there was a group of ten (10) elderly family caregivers who take care of an elderly person at home. The caregivers may or may not have been registered and/or monitored by the health teams of the municipality's Primary Health Care Units. The inclusion criteria for the elderly caregivers studied were: being over 60 years old and living in the area covered by primary health care units in the municipality of Juiz de Fora (MG).

At the time of the survey, the interviewees had to be lucid, oriented and aware; play the role of (main) family caregiver, i.e. have a family relationship with the elderly person: being a wife/husband/partner, child, daughter-in-law/son-in-law, sibling, living with the elderly person and being responsible for their care, regardless of ethnicity, color, religion, political position; and manifesting, in front of the researcher, that they are directly responsible for the care of a dependent elderly person, accepting to participate as unpaid volunteers, expressing their consent by signing the Informed Consent Form (ICF) (Appendix C).

4.2.3 Data collection

Data collection took place from August 2014 to January 2015 and began in the Primary Health Care Units located in the Nova Era and Santa Cruz neighborhoods, as they are the most populous neighborhoods in the northern region of the city, according to the Municipal Health Plan (JUIZ DE FORA, 2014c) and have ESFs. On the first visit, the nurse or manager of the unit was identified, explaining the purpose of the research and thus gaining access to information about the elderly living in the area covered by the Family Health Teams. The Community Health Agent (CHA) was then asked to accompany them on home visits, as a guarantee of the elderly's acceptance and reliability. It took an average of two visits to contact the nurses at each unit and then the CHW. The CHWs were chosen on the recommendation of the nurse, who indicated which areas the CHW was responsible for, taking into account the existence of elderly caregivers, in order to follow the criteria for inclusion in the study.

On a subsequent visit, CHWs who knew the micro-area for which they were responsible intentionally pointed out to me the families with elderly people who depended on being cared for at home by an elderly family caregiver. I was welcomed by the professionals, who readily agreed to accompany me on a first home visit (HV) to identify the family, introduce the researcher and the research. We then began to make appointments for subsequent data collection visits, according to the availability of each community worker and during working hours.

From there, the setting became the elderly person's home, and a home visit was adopted as the strategy for data collection. The aim of the HV was to get to know and characterize the elderly caregiver by conducting a semi-structured interview (APPENDIX D), observing and recording memos with the elderly caregivers who agreed to take part in the research, as previously agreed between the participant and the researcher.

Of the total number of participants, six agreed to take part on the first visit and four were quick to do so, but asked to call and make an appointment, as they couldn't at the time; no guest refused to take part in the research. The CHWs were asked to accompany the elderly during four visits in order to facilitate the data collection process, given the need for someone to remain with the elderly person during the interview with the caregiver. In three cases, the presence of the CHW was not necessary during the interview, as they left after the researcher was introduced. And in the last three interviews, the caregivers were identified through referrals from strangers in neighborhood stores, so there was no intermediation by a UAPS or monitoring by a CHA.

When it came to collecting empirical data on the TFD, the in-depth interview followed a line of dialogue between the interviewer and the interviewee. As the answers to the research questions emerged, others emerged. In addition to the data obtained from the interview, as described above, I used observation during each home visit. The field diary was written up immediately after the observation, on the interviewee's street or, if not, on the same day. This avoided the risk of missing any details.

During the home visit, it was observed that the caregivers were preparing for the interview, when it had been scheduled in advance, and that the presence of the researcher brought extreme comfort and relief to the caregivers. The satisfaction they showed in talking to someone, being listened to attentively, without rushing, left them free to talk about such everyday matters and sometimes so heavy to carry through life without being able to share. They showed great satisfaction at the simple fact of having someone to listen to them, and this was true in general, regardless of their financial situation. They all showed receptivity and gratitude and ended up asking me to come back more often, as I would be very welcome, thus confirming the importance of interpersonal relationships, especially through therapeutic listening.

Each visit lasted an average of an hour and a half to two hours, always concluding with a recorded interview, guided by the script. Before each interview, the ICF was read out to each participant, who then signed it and kept one copy. The field notes taken during the interviews were later better described and expanded.

The digital interviews were transcribed and the pre-analysis took place after the notes had been expanded and before the next visit, in accordance with Strauss and Corbin (2008). Based on the vision of Glaser and Straus (1967, p. 85), cited above, and based on the idea of the generating question, the instrument was restructured, allowing for a more flexible and comprehensive exposition of the topic, with the aim of delving deeper into the reality investigated and confirming the central category, with a view to validating the theoretical model.

During this phase, three more interviews were conducted with elderly caregivers from other neighborhoods: Benfica and Bairro Industrial, which still work with traditional health teams. At this stage, the approach to possible participants was based on referrals from unknown people, at commercial outlets such as clothing stores and beauty salons, where the researcher approached the professionals, asking if they knew anyone who met the inclusion criteria for the study. Now, however, I wanted the potential interviewees to have better financial conditions, in order to assess whether the issue of spirituality changed according to the socio-cultural and financial level of the individuals. From then on, I would visit the homes, explaining the purpose of the research and inviting them to take part in an interview. As before, they all accepted. I then scheduled the interviews according to their availability. At this stage, the process took place without the assistance of other health professionals.

For the textual editing of the empirical data, *software* was used, the OpenLogos program, version 1.0.2, due to the need to systematize the data from the extensive, unstructured texts originating from the transcriptions of the interviews, participant observation and notes recorded in a field diary. All the information was associated and worked on within the categories of analysis and grouped into the various passages identified, according to similarity.

OpenLogos is a textual data manager, developed by Kenneth Rochel de Camargo Júnior, with the function of storing and organizing data for analysis in a database (CAMARGO JUNIOR, 2003), which is a file with a standard "txt" extension. The program also allows a short descriptive text to be associated with each database and also generates a table of categories that can be used to mark segments of text, according to the user's interpretative criteria. Each category is identified by a code and a definition text, and the table is sorted alphabetically by code. A third table maintains the relationship between the categories and the documents, allowing them to be retrieved based on search criteria. The program also generates another table with a list of all the words that occur in the database in use, to be used later in the tabulation (CAMARGO JUNIOR, 2003).

OpenLogos allows you to manage an indefinite number of databases, each registered in a specific file on your computer's hard disk. This program is available free of charge to researchers who wish to use it (CAMARGO JUNIOR, 2003).

Inserting all the data generated into the program allowed it to be organized and then analyzed line by line, paragraph by paragraph, with each fragment that exposed a phenomenon being defined and coded with a term that represented it.

4.2.4 Ethical care

This research complied with the norms for Research with Human Beings, according to CNS Resolution 466/2012, which incorporates the four basic references of bioethics from the perspective of the individual and the collective: autonomy, non-maleficence, beneficence and justice. The document aims to guarantee the rights and duties of the scientific community, research participants and the State (BRASIL, 2012). In this sense, an ICF was drawn up to authorize the voluntary participation of the research subjects in the proposed care and for the interview. This form, which was signed by all those who agreed to take part in the study, describes the aim of the research and the entire process involved in carrying it out.

Participants were treated with dignity, with respect for their autonomy and vulnerability, as well as their cultural, social, moral, religious and ethical values in the research. Considering that all research involving human beings presents risks, we sought to weigh up the risks and benefits, both known and potential, individual and collective, assuming the commitment to obtain the maximum benefits and the minimum damage and risks. Data collection took place after the project had been approved by the Research Ethics Committee of the University Hospital of the Federal University of Juiz de Fora, according to a substantiated opinion published on the BRASIL Platform, number 676.364, on 26/05/2014 (Annex A).

To guarantee anonymity and preserve the identity of the participants, the names of the elderly caregivers have been replaced by biblical names, and there is no analogy with their first names.

According to the guidelines of the aforementioned resolution, the material recorded during data collection, the informed consent forms and all the data gathered in a physical or digital file during the research will be kept under the responsibility of the research coordinator for a period of five years and will then be destroyed in an appropriate manner. In addition, the results of the research, once finalized, will be made available to the participants and institutions involved and will be forwarded for publication (BRASIL, 2012).

5. THE LIFE CONTEXT OF ELDERLY CARERS IN THE PROCESS OF CARING FOR ANOTHER ELDERLY IN THE HOME AND THEIR CHALLENGES - ANALYSIS AND DISCUSSION

Let's take care of our hearts, because that's where the good and the bad come from, what builds and destroys.

Pope Francis

5.1 CHARACTERIZATION OF ELDERLY CAREGIVERS

What follows is an understanding of the life context and challenges faced by elderly family caregivers during the process of caring for others at home. The table is the result of an analysis of the empirical data collected from elderly family caregivers.

Table 1 shows the characterization of the elderly caregivers who took part in the study.

TABLE 1 - Identification of the elderly family caregivers of the elderly, with their respective elderly care dependents, participating in the research, by individual characteristics. Juiz de Fora - MG, 2015.

N.°	Identification of the main caregiver	Gender	Caregiver's current age	Marital relationship	Degree of kinship with the person being cared for	Identification of the person being cared for	Age	Core Family	Religious affiliation	Personal income
01	Adameire	Fem.	90 years	Married	Wife and mother	Jeremiah Sarah	93 years old 67 years old	Husband and two daughters	Non-practicing Spiritist	No income of their own
02	Isabel	Fem.	60 years old	Vihva	Daughter	Jesebel	93 years old	Màe	Catholic	Pensioner
03	Dina	Fem.	61 years old	Divorced	Daughter	Débora	86 years old	Màe	Non-practicing Catholic	Retired
04	Lia	Fem.	60 years old	Divorced	Daughter and sister	Maria Lucas	94 years old	Mother, brother and	Non-practicing Catholic	No income of their

							57 years old	daughter		own
05	Joshua	Fem.	70 years old	Married	Daughter	Gabriel	93 years old	Husband and father	Catholic	Retired
06	Gedeao	Male	61 years old	Married	Spouse	Ester	74 years old	Wife	Evangelical	Retired
07	Talita	Fem.	79 years old	Married	Wife	Emanuel	81 years old	Wife and daughter	Catholic	Retired
08	Ruth	Fem.	66 years	Married	Wife	Matthew	86 years old	Spouse and stepson	Evangelical	Retired
09	Samuel	Male	79 years old	Married	Spouse	Rebeca	74 years old	Wife	Catholic	Retired
10	Eunice	Fem.	73 years old	Married	Wife	Matthew	82 years old	Spouse	Non-practicing evangelical	Retired

According to chart 1, the focus group of the research was made up of ten elderly caregivers, the majority of whom were women, including wives and daughters, corroborating studies that indicate that women are the main caregivers. Ages ranged from 60 to 90 and most of the caregivers lived with partners. There were cases in which the caregiver was responsible for the care of more than one person, and this second person could be elderly or not. With regard to the age of the person being cared for, the majority are over 80. The income of most caregivers is due to retirement or pension, but there are cases of people who have no personal income at all, and are dependent on their children or the family member they care for. A relevant fact is that all caregivers have at least one chronic non-communicable disease (CNCD).

5.2 . PRESENTING CAREGIVERS IN THEIR DAILY LIVES

Taking the researcher's field diary records and observation notes as a reference, the following is a brief characterization of the life context of the main elderly caregivers who took part in the study, as listed in Table 1. It should be noted that when mentioning the name of each participant, a phrase expressing the essence of each caregiver, according to what was learned by the researcher during the visits and interviews, is included alongside.

5.2.1 Adameire - "Resilience in her daily struggle to promote the care of her daughter and husband".

The first home visit (HV 01) was to the house of Adameire, 90 years old, non-apparent. Born in Muriaé, she has dark brown skin, short stature, is slim, has brown eyes, short gray hair. The carer wears glasses and was wearing brown pants and a gray blouse, with black sandals open at the back. She appeared to be a person of total simplicity, with no adornments or painted nails. I was greeted with a shy smile on my face, but her countenance showed a certain sadness that, initially, I didn't declare.

The elderly woman lives on a seemingly quiet street, with a predominance of low-rise structures and large plots of land. She lives with her husband and two daughters on the first floor of a two-storey house with old paintwork. I entered through a small gray door next to the garage. According to the interviewee, upstairs lives her daughter-in-law, who is separated from her son and, even after the marital break-up, the two have a good relationship. The house looked clean; as we entered the kitchen, there were clothes on the table, and I was told by the elderly woman that she was collecting the clothes from the clothesline and folding them. She then took the opportunity to say that she did all the housework, except cleaning and ironing, because she said she feels "a lot of pain in her body, her blood pressure rises sometimes, and it's not like it used to be".

She talked well, telling us everything in great detail. Her appearance was rather haggard, with sad eyes, in keeping with her difficult life story: the mother of six children, including a lawyer, a federal tax auditor and a physiotherapist, she was weighed down by the burden of looking after her 69-year-old daughter (Sarah), who, according to Adameire, was born with cerebral palsy and is, as far as I could tell, totally dependent, babbling a few words with difficulty, standing up only with help. The only reason Adameire isn't bathing her daughter is that she pays a girl to do it. However, the interviewee is not very happy about this, as she says that "she [the helper] doesn't bathe her properly" and that she has to stay with her, taking care of her.

Ademeire also takes care of her husband, Mr. Jeremias, her second marriage, to whom she has been married for over 60 years. Her husband is 93 years old, black, tall and has sequelae from the stroke he suffered in 1995; he is currently diagnosed with advanced prostate cancer (according to Adameire). He walks around pushing a simple kitchen chair, as if it were a walker and, as far as I could tell, with a high risk of falling, because the wooden planks were coming loose and Adameire herself complained that it was dangerous and that she had also fallen many times because of the "bumpy" floor. She said that she bathes her husband because he can't do it on his own, but she finds it very difficult and insecure to do so because he is very tall and she is so short, and he can't sit up because of swelling in his genital area (not seen). She said that she is afraid that he will fall and that this is what makes her most insecure in her daily care.

In her speech, Adameire showed a certain bitterness towards her daughter, who is well-off, because she feels she needs support to carry out her caring role. This became clear when she said that neither she nor Sarah have retired to this day, because her daughter has made them "her dependents" and, as a result, the elderly woman can't buy anything, nor can she fix the floor. She also said that her daughter pays for her health insurance and does the shopping, but sometimes it's not enough, because she doesn't have the freedom to buy anything: "The money from his pension is barely enough to buy the medicines, which are very expensive."

Adameire said she loved reading and that it brought her comfort and well-being, and that she read every night. She showed a mixture of emotions during the interview: she cried, her voice was often hoarse, she showed sadness, she said she was afraid of dying because of her daughter, who was totally dependent on her care.

With resignation, she assures us that, regardless of her religion (she has been a Spiritualist for 62 years, but stopped attending five years ago due to the overload of daily work and because she had no one to leave her husband and daughter with when she left home), she believes that her strength comes from God, as she said: "I don't take a drop of water at dawn before thanking God for everything, as well as asking for the strength to continue on my way". She made a point of showing the books (from Seicho-no-ie) that she likes to read and which, according to her, give her the strength to continue on her path. She also said that she "listens to the Bible on cassette tapes that her daughter gave her".

I noticed that she felt extremely grateful for the opportunity to speak freely and to have someone listen to her, without judgment or impositions, just listening to her life story. Adameire said goodbye with a big hug, a lighter countenance, thanked me very much and asked me to come back more often, demonstrating the importance of the interpersonal relationship between the health professional and the client.

5.2.2 Isabel - "A story of love and resignation".

The second home visit (HV 02) was to the home of Isabel, 60, from the town of Tabuleiro (MG), who had been widowed for two years. She is white, short, has light, short hair, green eyes and is the mother of three children. She welcomed me wearing a brown long-sleeved blouse, sweatpants and black open-toed sandals. I was greeted with a warm hug.

The elderly woman lives with her mother in a wide, paved street, with a predominance of low, not fully built houses, close to the square and the church. The street is located in the lower part of the neighborhood and does not present any difficulties in terms of access. The elderly woman's house has two floors, with her home on the first and one of her daughters on the top. The other daughter lives across the street from her house. When I entered the house, I couldn't help but notice how zealously she takes care of the upkeep, how clean everything is, and how the living room is a small place with lots of religious and family photos. The house is well maintained and has treated water and a sewage system.

Isabel told us how she began to look after her mother, who is now 93, showing great calm and satisfaction with the life she leads; she stressed at all times the importance of the support of her family (daughters and brothers), making it clear that she loves life and that her strength to go on each day comes from God and that without this strength nothing would be possible. She showed herself to be a very religious person, active in the Catholic religion and who goes to Mass every week when one of her siblings stays with their mother.

Finally, Isabel showed no difficulties in caring for her mother, who appeared to be very well cared for, or in self-care, and she also reported that she had been practicing water aerobics for almost a year, while her daughter, who lives across the street, remained with her grandmother. At no point did the interviewee feel alone and she reports that she has the support of the team at the Primary Care Unit, including the ACS, doctor and nurse. She said she liked the idea of having someone from the health sector at home to answer her questions and find out about her illnesses: hypertension and rheumatoid arthritis.

5.2.3 Dina - "Giving up one's life for the sake of caring".

The third home visit (HV 03) was to the home of Dina, from Juiz de Fora (MG), divorced, 61 years old, white, short, with dark brown hair below her shoulders and brown eyes, mother of three children. She greeted me wearing a gray blouse under a black cold coat and black shorts with white stripes down the sides, below her knees; she was wearing golden slippers.

I arrived at her home accompanied by the Community Health Agent responsible for that area. It's worth emphasizing that I was surprised by the affection, politeness and respect he showed the users, and I took the opportunity to give him some advice, showing great solicitude and availability if necessary. I was greeted with a warm hug, a smile on my face and a gratifying politeness.

Dina lives on a paved street, where small and medium-sized buildings are mixed with many one- and two-storey houses. Nearby I could see an evangelical church. The street is located in the moderately uphill part of the neighborhood, but there are no difficulties in accessing it. The interviewee lives in a four-storey building, but her home is on the second floor and is accessed via a corridor, with no stairs.

As soon as I entered her home, I could *already* see that it was hygienic and that the apartment was medium-sized and airy, thanks to a balcony in the living room. On the small bookshelf, photos of family members were scattered around, demonstrating her attachment to her family, which could also be seen in her speech. The apartment is rented, and she has only been living in the neighborhood for two months, as she has her own house in a nearby neighborhood. However, Dina told me that she has been taking care of her children since she decided to look after her mother and ended up leaving everything behind. She also told me that there are lots of dogs in her house, which her mother doesn't like. Dina currently lives with her mother, whom she looks after, and two of her children, her eldest daughter and her youngest son.

The interviewee showed at all times that the interview was for her to vent and she seemed grateful that I was there, allowing her to tell me her story. She told me how she began to take full care of her mother, who is now 86, more than two years ago and that this resulted in some family disagreements with seven siblings, including her. When she told me about when she decided to take care of her mother, who at the time lived with another sister in another part of the city, she expressed herself carefully, showing that her speech was not intended to denigrate her sister's image, but rather to show the reason for her action.

She reported, with a certain sadness, that when she came to visit her mother, she smelled bad (urine) and she could see that her mother wasn't eating properly. What was most striking was that when she visited her mother, she wouldn't accept her leaving at the end of the day. The whole family disagreement, the revolt of all the siblings was, according to the interviewee, "because they thought she wanted to take advantage of her mother's pensions", one of which was her mother's personal pension for length of service and the pension she received from her deceased husband. The situation seems to have had a negative impact on Mrs. Dina who, at all times, showed sadness and emotion when she spoke, especially when she said that "at first all the siblings stayed away, no one went to visit them".

Anyway, today, as she says: "they have come to realize that I just wanted to take care of her and, every day that they see their mother, they say that she is well, smelling good and well cared for". She went on to say: "my greatest sadness is that one of my siblings, with whom I was closest, has moved away and since then has never come to see me, and won't even look at me". At every moment of the interview, I realized that this is a distressing issue for the interviewee, one that causes her worry and sadness, affecting her more than the change of life itself, to the detriment of the act of caring for a person as a whole, which has undoubtedly corroborated several changes in her daily life.

Dina does all the housework and says she is very homely, showing calm and satisfaction with the life she leads, even with the difficulties she faces all the time. She shows that she seeks relief in "a higher being", who gives her the strength to live and continue with her task as a caregiver, strength that made her overcome the clashes caused by her family when she decided to take on the task of caring and give up so many things in her life. To relax and relieve tension, she says she likes to listen to music from different genres, such as gospel and country, and watch soap operas on TV.

She showed that she is a spiritual person, that she is Catholic, but that lately, before the move, she had been attending an evangelical church, because she said that her brother baptized her mother in his church and, as she doesn't go out without her and doesn't want to cause "confusion" by taking her mother to a Catholic church, she prefers to go to the evangelical church herself. At this point, she once again demonstrated her spirituality, present and giving her strength at all times to keep going. Her speech showed how she believes in a higher being who, in her view, is God, who gives strength and encouragement, regardless of religion. So much so that she says she is not attending any church at the moment, but that she does intend to look for one that is easier, due to the difficulty of leaving the house, as her mother can't walk very far and she doesn't have her own car.

She claimed that she couldn't talk in detail about the primary care team that assists her, given the short time she's been living in the neighborhood, but said that the health agent is very friendly and that her mother also likes him a lot.

As for her state of health, she said that she suffers from hypertension, which is controlled, and is living with a possible diagnosis of fibromyalgia. When we said goodbye, she and her mother took me to the exit door, we talked a lot and she thanked me sincerely, invited me to come back and again spoke of God and her belief in his power. She also believes in the importance of forgiveness, because she knows that everything will work out and, even though she believes she hasn't done anything wrong against her brother, she wants to ask him for forgiveness. Again, she insisted that I come back and said goodbye, telling me to go with God and that she sincerely hoped she had contributed to my work.

5.2.4 Lia - "Attributing all her strength to the divine: physical and emotional overload influenced by a lack of family support".

The fourth home visit (HV 04) was to the home of Lia, 60, from Urucânia, near Ponte Nova

(MG). The mother of two daughters, one married and the other aged 13, Lia is divorced and currently lives with her youngest daughter, her brother and her mother, the latter two being her main and, one might say, only carers. The former is 58 years old and has a mental disorder and has always required special care; the latter, who is 94, is in a state of total dependence.

When we arrived at her house with the CHA responsible for the area, we were greeted by the interviewee in a warm and receptive manner. She invited us into her house, which had a small living room with the two family members she cares for. Her brother was lying on a small two-seater sofa and watching television; her mother was on the other sofa, with her eyes closed, looking pained.

I was invited by Lia to go into the kitchen so that "we could talk more freely". Her house is quite simple and is on a lower level than the street, which makes it difficult to access, as there are some steps, which are a bit steep, especially when it comes to taking her mother out for a walk or even when she needs to go out with her for any reason.

Lia is a woman of medium height, with brown eyes, fair skin, straight brown hair, with a few white strands that were tied up in an unruly tail. She was wearing lead-colored knitted shorts below her knees, an aged light green knitted blouse, very old sandals, no ornaments and her toenails had worn off. Her countenance showed no joy. On the contrary, I noticed that her eyes were sad, which I was able to understand during the interview.

The caregiver lives in a neighborhood in the city that has a mixture of accentuated poverty and middle and upper-middle class. Her street is located in the upper part of the neighborhood, on a hill, in one of the most deprived areas of the neighborhood. The street is made up of many low, simple houses and, at the back of her house, there is a small house (not shown) where, according to Lia, her eldest daughter, who has just had a baby, currently lives.

Her house is moderately clean, and Lia is responsible for all the household chores, but she says that "it's hard to keep everything clean", both because she depends on her mother and because of her mother's preoccupation with cleaning. According to Lia, her mother "always fights" when she starts cleaning, so she has to do everything little by little. Her mother really depends on her caregiver in every way, for both BADL and IADL tasks, for example: she can't walk, dress or bathe herself, and even eating is proving difficult. Her mother was lying down the whole time I was at her home and spoke very little. Except when we were in the kitchen during the interview and, because Lia had "disappeared", she started calling her by name, insistently, proving how the caregiver creates an almost exclusive bond with the caregiver, which often prevents them from carrying out other activities.

One aspect that I considered relevant, considering the question of this research, and again emphasized by the caregiver, was the spiritual side, which even moved me during the interview. It was important to see how people seek strength in a higher being, "God", who, regardless of religion, sustains them on a daily basis, giving them the strength to overcome life's obstacles which, in the case of this interviewee, are not few, among them: the lack of family support, financial dependence, the lack of a partner and the daily care of her mother, who is totally dependent, her brother and a teenage daughter. She showed herself to be a person extremely lacking in affection, alone and with few possibilities for self-care. She says that she is "going through a very heavy phase", as she has no support from her other siblings, and she cried a lot during the interview, showing a deep sense of sadness and abandonment.

Once again, I realized that caregivers feel respected and grateful when we stop to listen to them, even if we don't intervene, except to actively listen to their entire life story. They show that, often, this is even more important than carrying out direct health care (procedures). Lia asked me to come back again, because no one had ever stopped to listen to her or her feelings.

5.2.5 Joshua - "Religiosity as a major force, combined with the Companionship of the husband: life story as a caregiver".

The fifth home visit (HV 05) was to the home of Joshua, 70 years old, from Piedade do Rio Grande (MG), mother of 4 children (one of whom died five years ago of chronic kidney disease). When we arrived at her house with the CHA responsible for the area, we were greeted by her husband, a very nice man, who welcomed us with a smile on his face, showing a lot of sympathy and, as soon as he invited us in, we were already in his living room.

I was struck by the cleanliness and also the decoration, with several pictures of Jesus and some images of saints on the walls. The room was very bright and airy.

Next came Joshua, dark-skinned, short, weighing in line with his height, with brown eyes, black hair with gray roots, unpainted, tied back in a ponytail. She was wearing black pants and a black and white printed blouse, with a thin white belt around her waist, black sandals, open at the back, and prescription glasses, very simply, she didn't have any adornments, nor were her nails painted. She welcomed us well and her countenance showed serenity, which was proven during the interview.

Joshua, his husband and her father, a 93-year-old man, live in an apparently quiet street, with buildings and many beautiful houses around, and a bus stop opposite. The family lives in a nice house with a terrace; the paintwork, green in color, looks new, with a fence and a good number of plants. The space also includes a house at the back (not shown), where the 47-year-old son lives alone. According to the elderly, "he's an alcoholic" and used to live in another neighborhood, in his own house, but because of his problem and because he doesn't take care of himself properly, they convinced him to move in with them. Joshua's house looks very clean and she assures me that she is responsible for all the household chores, but that she has her husband on whom she can always rely. I could tell, from the way they looked at each other, the way they talked and even from the husband's participation in the interview, that they share a unique complicity.

They have been together for 55 years and, surely, part of the interviewee's apparent serenity, despite all the tasks and responsibilities of being the main caregiver, is due to this union. The other part comes from her developed religiosity/spirituality, which is demonstrated at all times in her speech. Joshua reported that he has some health problems, but at no point did he complain or at least show any kind of suffering or overload due to the act of caring.

She spoke well, recounting everything in great detail; she showed a certain amount of apprehension in a certain question, in terms of feelings of tension and anguish, because the question referred to the possibility of her dying and, if this happened, what would become of her father and her husband? At this point, the husband also intervened, saying that "neither of them can be without the other, because they have always helped each other and intend to continue that way". At the end of the interview, I was able to meet his father, who was resting and, according to Joshua, has a listening deficit. He seemed to be very "playful", a gentleman with a good appearance, certainly with impeccable hygiene.

The elderly woman emphasized that she has a very large family, spread across Volta Redonda, Barbacena, Piedade, Sao Joao Del Rey, but the couple remembered the importance of their daughter who died and was undergoing hemodialysis, who "God took away". She was very close to her grandfather and therefore helped a lot, because when the couple wanted to go out, even when the daughter was already undergoing hemodialysis, she would stay with her grandfather. This made the couple's relationship easier, because they were able to go out together more and, as I noticed, this is a crucial point, because they had always been close, they liked to "go out and travel together", because now they don't do it anymore. They repeated several times during the interview how much they miss their daughter. What caught my attention during the interview was the couple's complicity and Joshua's developed spirituality/religiosity which, once again, demonstrated the importance of working on the spiritual dimension in order to achieve comprehensive, quality care. Another point is the link between the family and the CHW, which should also be developed by the nurse. It was clear that they were grateful for the visit, were very pleasant and told us to come back more often.

5.2.6 Gedeao - "Owner of an unshakeable faith that gives him security for life and the process of caring for others"

The sixth home visit (HV 06) was to the home of Gedeao, 61, who cares for his wife, Ester, 74, to whom he has been married for seven years. She is diabetic and as a result had to have the lower part of her left limb amputated. They live in a paved, flat street in the lower part of the neighborhood. The surrounding houses were as simple as the couple's, which is not their own, having been rented out four years ago when the wife had her limb amputated. Before, they lived with Esther's daughter, but "it didn't work out", according to Gedeao. They lead a simple life and get by on their pensions. Gedeao says he is responsible for all the household chores and also for taking his wife to the doctor, for check-ups or follow-ups at ACISPES[2] and at the neighborhood Primary Health Care Unit.

They are both evangelicals and regularly attend church, where he takes her in her wheelchair. The house seems to be small, although I haven't seen all of it, I've only seen the living room and the couple's bedroom. When we arrived at his house (the ACS and I), Gedeao greeted us politely, asking us to wait a while as he was helping his wife to shower. After a few minutes, he left her in the bedroom and came to see us, apologizing. He said that he would help her shower, but that she would change herself.

Gedeao was wearing burgundy shorts, a beige T-shirt and flip-flops. He looks good and is fit; he's tall, dark, has slightly graying hair and a neat beard. He told me about the responsibility of looking after him, but that even so, "he thanks God every morning for giving him the strength to carry on". And when he feels down, God renews him, so he said that "the love that God has for us is gratifying". He also says that he finds it difficult because "he looks after it alone", since his wife's daughter hardly ever comes, so "wherever he goes he has to take Ester". He shows a lot of concern for his own health, as he says he "has to be on his feet to look after her", so he tries to look after himself. When asked about medical appointments, such as a urologist, cardiologist or preventive tests such as prostate cancer, he said that he "goes every year" and also has a prostate ultrasound. But he takes his wife with him, because he can't leave her alone either.

One difficulty he felt and reported was in terms of accessibility, since every day he is faced with a lack of access, for example, "a lack of bus stops to make it easier". He said that these are things that sadden him, because they don't only happen to him. Then he brings God into

---

2 The Agência de Cooperaçao Intermunicipal em Saùde Pè da Serra (ACISPES) is a non-profit civil association based in Juiz de Fora, Minas Gerais, created in 1996; it is a consortium of 24 municipalities whose focus is health promotion, with the provision of medium-complexity consultations and exams and transportation for patients. Available at: http://www.acispes.co m.br/?pagina=quem.

the conversation and says that God says to him: "Son, I'm giving you strength, keep going, then continue on your way without getting discouraged". He shows great confidence in carrying out the care, because he is driven by God. The question is how to organize yourself to be able to carry out all the activities and also take care of yourself.

To relieve daily tensions, he says he likes to "sing praises and read the Bible. Then the sadness goes away". It was a very rich interview, he showed himself to be a wise person, focused on his goals and with a very developed spirituality/religiosity. He thanked us for the conversation which, according to him, "was very rich and healthy" and said: "it's very good to see that someone cares about us, listens to us and helps us solve our problems". He closed by saying that "the gospel is not a religion, it leads to only one path: God".

5.2.7 Talita - "God's strength to go on, always".

The seventh home visit (HV 07) was to the home of Talita, 79, the mother of seven children, six of whom are married and a single woman who lives with the couple and is a manicurist. They live on a very busy street, as it is one of the main ones in the neighborhood, which is paved and located in a flat area, with easy access, with the presence of buildings and many houses, as well as a variety of shops. Arriving with the ACS was interesting, as Mrs. Talita has a habit of tying the key to a rope and throwing it to those who arrive, so that they don't have to go down the stairs, and the ACS told me that she is already used to the procedure. We opened a door, which gave access to a staircase with two small flights, each with six steps, but steep, and the staircase was very narrow, which seemed to make it difficult to pass, especially with a wheelchair.

At the end of the stairs, we came to a huge, airy and comfortable balcony, where we found the couple. Mr. Emanuel, looking well-groomed, was sitting comfortably in a chair, with a walking stick leaning against his side, and could see every movement in the street. Dona Talita came to meet us with a big smile and already commented on the heat, which was very hot. She is a white lady, of medium height, apparently overweight, with straight, short, black hair tied back behind her ears, with a few white roots to be touched up, and brown eyes.

She greeted me wearing a loose-fitting, knee-length T-shirt with a red and white floral print and comfortable black flip-flops that covered the front of her feet and were open at the back; she wore prescription glasses and didn't wear much adornment, just a small transparent stone earring; her nails were unpainted; she looked well-groomed. She was cordial and interested in taking part in the study. The interview took place on her balcony and, although I didn't enter her house, it seemed large and clean. They own their home and the downstairs has a garage, a sewing studio and an extra room for their daughter to work in. The couple are retired, she used to work as a seamstress and her husband was a shopkeeper. They seem to have a quiet life in terms of their financial situation, they have health insurance and generally use it for consultations, exams, etc. They don't use the services of the primary health care unit, but she said that she has already received visits from the doctor and always receives the ACS; she only feels that she can't receive medicines from the UAPS and has to buy them every month because she can't pick them up (the UAPS is very far from her house).

D. Talita has shown that she is confident and determined in her life and says that she is that way because of God's strength. She said that "the task of caring is not easy and only those who feel it on their skin know what it's like". She has been the main caregiver for over thirty years, as she said, since her husband had his first stroke. She emphasized that she has no one to replace her in the care routine, except in sporadic cases. She told me that she has "several problems" with her health and showed me her feet, which are deformed as a result of the arthritis that has been with her for some years and which makes her feel "terrible pain, which no longer goes away with the use of common painkillers", quoting the name of a more powerful drug. She also suffers from hypertension, hemorrhoids, diverticulitis and reflux. However, she said that she "remains firm", always feeding her belief which, according to her, makes her continue to live and take care of herself.

At times during the interview, her eyes would glaze over and fill with tears, and she would say that "her relief comes from God", through her prayers. She also said that she often goes into her room and cries a lot, as a way of letting off steam, because she misses someone to listen to her and understand her. Once again, I was struck by the strength that this caregiver showed, affirming at various times that everything is only possible through belief, through spiritual searching, through her faith in God.

5.2.8 Ruth - "Facing challenges and adaptations to her own aging, firm in her religious beliefs to take care of a dependent family member."

The eighth home visit (HV 08) took place at the home of Ruth, born in Juiz de Fora, married, 66 years old, black, apparently overweight, short, with dark hair and eyes. She has no natural children, but says she has six stepchildren who are real gifts from God. She welcomed me wearing a printed blouse with a white background and a red skirt, with simple, comfortable-looking shoes. I was greeted with a warm hug.

The lady lives in a well-located, easily accessible, paved street, made up of low-rise houses, two buildings, a bazaar which, by the way, belongs to her stepdaughter, a bakery and a glass shop. Her house was the last on a long plot of land, and I passed through a small gate that gave access to a wide corridor where there were several of the family's houses. Her house was simple, easily accessible and hygienic, and Ruth said that she was the one who did all the daily chores, "thank God". She seemed very comfortable telling me about her life and spoke with a twinkle in her eye, with great joy for her family and her six stepchildren.

In her speech, she demonstrated that her foundation at all times and for everything in her life, the support and sustenance for the task of caring for her husband on a daily basis, is "in the first place, the strength of God and, secondly, her family". Mr. Mateus, her husband, has sequelae from the stroke he suffered in 1996 and she says that he was in a serious condition, having even been "discouraged" by the doctor. After his recovery, which was considered a miracle, he spent a long time in a local hospital until he was able to return home and, from then on, she never stopped looking after him. She said that, for the last year, "he's gotten a lot worse", "he's even started drooling". However, she maintains her strength, even though she feels a lot of "pain in her legs", caused by arthritis, and says that, despite all the difficulty her husband has walking, "he doesn't sit still", which puts a lot of strain on her, because she's afraid to leave him alone, because he wouldn't either: "he's afraid of getting sick alone, for example. If he's lying down and alone, he won't be able to get up." She said that she always tries to be there and that she "bathes him, does everything", but sometimes he stays with his stepdaughter so that she can rest a bit during the day, especially when she's in a lot of pain.

Ruth showed herself to be an extremely religious, practicing person, currently an evangelical, but she said that for many years she was a Catholic. She firmly believes in overcoming life's adversities through faith. She doesn't receive institutionalized support for the daily care of her husband and uses the private network for his health care and her own. Once again, what caught my attention during the visit and interview was the great strength she shows through her faith in God, thanking Him for everything and, at all times and with the support of her family, ensuring that the caregiver is able to follow her path with less burden. When she left, she said that she had been prepared for caring since she was young, when she cared for three people, one blind, one mute and the other deaf. And yet, with God's help, she was always able to cope, in fact, she said: "God was preparing me".

5.2.9 Samuel - "Without God nothing is possible, with God everything will work out".

The ninth home visit (HV 09) was to the home of Samuel, 79, father of two daughters, married, one a teacher and the other a psychologist, one living in Juiz de Fora and the other in Brasilia, accompanying her husband, who is a manager at the Bank of Brazil. He is the grandfather of two granddaughters, two of whom live in Brasilia, one is a lawyer and the other is studying communications engineering, while the other, a doctor, is finishing a specialization course in Sao Paulo. He was very happy, excited and proud to talk about his daughters and, even more so, his granddaughters.

When I arrived at his house, I was greeted by him with great cordiality and respect. At this point, he made a comment and praised my punctuality, as I had booked the interview for 3pm by phone and arrived three minutes early. I could see that he was already waiting for me and, at that moment, he showed his concern for welcoming visitors.

Mr. Samuel has dark skin, brown eyes, short stature and is balding; he was wearing white shorts, a grey T-shirt and leather sandals, showing excellent hygiene. He and his wife live in an apparently quiet street, with a few buildings and lots of houses. I was soon invited inside, so we climbed two flights of stairs of about 12 steps each. Her house has three floors, the first of which is an apartment that is empty because they say that if they rent it out, they could lose their privacy, and a duplex on the second floor. When I entered her living room, I was struck by the cleanliness and the very tasteful decoration, with a large chandelier hanging in the living room, showing a certain sophistication, the lowered ceilings, the living room with two rooms, some extremely tasteful paintings, completing the decoration. The house is very bright and airy.

As soon as we entered, he took me to the bedroom where his wife, Rebeca, 74, was lying in bed, in a large, well-decorated and clean room, with exquisite curtains. You could see that they were well-off and had a very peaceful life. For some years now, Rebeca has been developing rheumatoid arthritis, a chronic and degenerative disease that has been progressively impeding her movement for the last four years. She walks with great difficulty, only from the bedroom to the bathroom, or to the kitchen for lunch, with the help of crutches and her husband. To get out of the house, she relies on crutches and wheelchairs. That doesn't stop her from being vain, looking great, with straight, black, shoulder-length hair that looked like it had just come out of a beauty salon. And, as she said, her hair is "always dyed, because, despite my woes, I like to take care of myself", and she added: "I like to take care of myself in every way, from hygiene and beauty care to food and health." Rebeca was covered in a white bedspread, with a huge fan on.

She said that she has a health insurance plan and prefers to use hospital care, outpatient care and tests in the private network (by private agreement). Her carer and husband, on the other hand, says he prefers to go to the UAPS, which doesn't have an ESF and works under the traditional model, where he gets his medication and is "very well looked after by everyone", leaving him to use the health insurance only in the case of exams and surgeries, "because it doesn't take long, since the SUS takes a long time". Rebeca is talkative and was very worried about her unfinished nails, because her manicurist, according to her, had traveled and so she hadn't been able to do her nails that week. Rebeca expresses herself well and says that she is retired and used to be a civil servant.

As previously mentioned, the house has two floors, the second of which is not visible, and is very clean, which is the responsibility of Mr. Samuel, who makes a point of saying that he takes care of it alone and that Rebekah is too demanding, has a mania for cleanliness and that they find it difficult to find trustworthy people, which is why he "prefers to manage on his own". The clothes are taken to a laundress and the food is bought, and he's only responsible for the small snacks, as it's difficult to do everything alone. That's why they chose to buy, not to mention that the restaurant has great food, with a varied menu. He also said that he likes Japanese food and, from time to time, a good wine. He says he loves cooking and knows how to make a variety of dishes, from the most sophisticated to the simplest, and likes to make "sweet pies and snacks with prawns".

According to the reports, they have been together for 57 years and show that they love and respect each other, treating each other with a lot of affection, but she made a point of saying that she is "very jealous". As in the other interviews, here the story repeats itself: the caregiver has health problems, takes antihypertensive medication and has a "problem" with his right knee, which is made difficult by the stairs. However, at no point did he complain or at least show any kind of suffering or overload as a result of the act of caring; on the contrary, I was surprised by his care for himself and his serenity in caring for his wife, all very safely.

Samuel vehemently affirms his conviction of God's presence in his life and claims that he has nothing to be thankful for. In fact, the only time he showed a certain amount of anxiety was about the possibility of something happening to him; he even showed that all the doors have a four-key, because if something happened to him, his wife would be protected until their daughter arrived. As for family support, they say that if they need it, they can count on their family, even though they are all busy; however, they showed a lot of independence, leaving family members to turn to only as a last resort. What struck me most during the visit and interview was the strength and spiritual quest emanating from both of them in that environment. She was fervent in her prayers, demonstrated through her speech and perceived by the presence of many images of Jesus and other saints of her devotion, alongside photos of the family.

Samuel, on the other hand, showed great serenity, patience, wisdom and reverence for God at all times, from my arrival to my departure from that home. He said he was "God-fearing", Catholic, but said he respected all religions, because they all seek God. He said he goes to Mass every week and watches TV, but he has an obligation to go to God's house, adding: "I have to dedicate part of my time to Him". Once again, I noticed that they were grateful for the visit and were very pleasant, saying that they would like to come back more often. The visit took three and a half hours, with a lot of talking and learning. The interview took place in a room, without his wife present.

5.2.10 Eunice - "Victorious because of her trust in God and love for her husband"

The tenth home visit (HV 10) was to the home of Eunice, a native of the municipality of Ponte Nova (MG), married, in her second marriage for twenty years, aged 73. I was greeted with a broad smile, her eyes are lively, showing great pleasure in life. She is white, short, overweight and has straight, short, light brown hair and honey-colored eyes. She welcomed me in a blouse and shorts set with a discreet print. She wore brown sandals open at the back and prescription glasses; simply put, she didn't have many adornments, just a small earring, her nails were painted and she looked great.

The mother of three daughters, one of whom was adopted, her husband actually "took her in to raise" and, when they got together, she took over the care of her daughter with him. As for her two biological daughters, one lives in Switzerland for work and the other lives in the city of Rio de Janeiro with her husband and children, where Eunice also lived for over 15 years and met her current "beloved husband", Mr. Mateus. Eunice lives on a paved street, where small and medium-sized buildings mix with many one-storey houses and duplexes. I noticed a Catholic church on the corner of her house. The street is located in one of the highest parts of the neighborhood, with a steep ascent, but it doesn't offer any difficulties in getting around, as the interviewee has her own vehicle and "drives everywhere", saying that she "decided to get her license after her husband went bad in 2000 and she had a lot of trouble sorting things out". She says that if she hadn't been licensed to drive, she wouldn't have known what to do.

She lives in her own large, airy house, which I could see was hygienic, clean and well decorated; it also has a library, which the interviewee made a point of showing me, as it contains several copies of the books her husband wrote. He, a retired lawyer, according to Eunice, was a writer, a journalist, "had an extremely active life", and showed himself to be cultured, as we talked from the moment I arrived until we left. Mrs. Eunice was proud of her husband and showed "unquestionable love for him", whom she took care of with love and patience. I could see her emotion at various moments during the interview. He was sitting on the sofa in the TV room, watching a program, while showing impeccable care, dressed in comfortable but refined pyjamas, with a clean shave and tidy hair.

Eunice told me that she started looking after her husband, who is now 82, in 2000, when he "had a stroke". However, after three months of rehabilitation, he was already driving, without any sequelae. From 2007 onwards, he began to have "a weakness in his legs, he would lock them, but he couldn't walk", and that's when they moved to their current address. In 2010, he had another "beginning of a stroke", then started having "episodes of labyrinthitis" and, from then on, he couldn't be left alone, "he can't go to the toilet on his own", he depends on care. She said that she lives for her husband and that she does this with a lot of love and care, because she "loves him too much". The interviewee verbalized the difficulty, given that she no longer has a social life, "he doesn't accept someone else to look after him", except when he needs to solve "some problem". Her adopted daughter, who lives in a nearby neighborhood, helps her whenever necessary.

At all times during the interview, she showed an "unshakeable faith", with a strength that, for her, undoubtedly "comes from God". The couple have an evangelical religious affiliation, but for some time now, they are no longer able to "attend services", but watch them on TV, because he can't bear to go and she won't leave him at home, she doesn't feel safe leaving him alone, she says she is "afraid that something bad will happen to him in her absence". She seeks moments of distraction on the computer, talking to her friends and her daughters.

She reported that she was the one who took care of her husband, including his beard, hair and nails. According to the interviewee, she has to "take special care" because he is diabetic. Eunice said that she does all the housework, but has a helper who helps her once a week, as the house is very large, with huge windows to clean. As for self-care, I noticed that she tries to go for routine check-ups and exams, taking advantage of the times when her husband also goes. They get all their care through private health insurance. She said that her husband had been admitted to hospital via SUS, but "regretted it bitterly" and from then on began to "pay for a complete plan for him and her to have private exams and consultations". When the carer needs her, the daughter stays with her father so that she can have some health check-ups, like going to the endocrinologist, because she discovered that she had a "thyroid problem" six years ago and has been taking medication ever since. Eunice is also diabetic, hypertensive and reports feeling "a lot of pain in her body", which started a year ago.

She was resistant to practicing physical activity, having already been told to walk or do aqua aerobics, but she still hasn't accepted, claiming that she "doesn't have the time". At all times during the interview, she showed great love for her husband, but what really struck me, as in all the other interviews, is how much they express their spirituality, with a mysterious strength and devotion, a daily and incessant search for divine graces, which is perceived by the confident and proper speech of the interviewees.

The caregiver only showed insecurity when talking about her death, which can be explained by the fact that she has to leave her husband, "and what would become of him?" One worry is imagining that he will have to live the rest of his life in a nursing home. Even so, she gets over her insecurity, based on her belief in God. According to her, it is He who strengthens her every day. Eunice, like the other participants, was grateful to have the opportunity to talk about her life and claimed that she "just keeps it all" and with me she felt at ease, she was able to open up and talk about what happens in her day-to-day life as her husband's main carer.

5.3 OPEN CODING

At this stage of the analysis, in which the empirical material can be coded into as many codes as possible (STRAUSS; CORBIN, 2008) and all the data can be coded at this stage of the analysis, we arrived at a set of 39 codes, which can be seen in TABLE 2:

TABLE 2- Open coding: generation of 39 codes related to the issue under investigation

N.θ	Empirical data - Excerpts from interviews with participants	Codes
1	*I started looking after him when he had a stroke in 96, my daughter. From then on, I started looking after him and, thank God, I still do today.* (Ruth)	Growing old and becoming the main family caregiver.
2	*I don't take a drop of water in the morning until I thank God: I thank him for my life, for the lives of my children and my husband. The house is in pieces, but it's mine, right? I give thanks by going! I believe that God is the one who gives strength to everyone, everything we go through is by his will. If we fail to understand or desire his presence with us, we have no life, our life is divine light. And God's strength."* (Adameire)	SpiritualityZreligiosity as strength and support for life.
3	*The difficulty is when it comes to bathing. (Isabel) Difficult. It's very complicated, you just have to live it day by day [to understand]. I have to give medicine in my hand, water in my hand, everything is in my hand. And he doesn't like accepting someone else either, it's difficult, complicated, and now it's getting worse, because his head is getting really bad; you've had three strokes, right? (Talita)*	Physical overload of the elderly caregiver's role.
4	*I have rheumatoid arthritis, [...] I have two prostheses, I can't walk."* (Isabel)	The compromised health of elderly caregivers.

	I have arthrosis in my feet, in my knees, I feel severe pain, [which] makes me almost unable to walk. There are days, to give you an idea, [that] I take tramadol, because I'm in so much pain. (Talita)	
5	*I have to do everything for her, I help her bathe, I'm afraid she'll fall. So even when I encourage her, I stand close by and hate it. I have to help eia get dressed, eia gets dressed, but because of her arm, because of the stroke, she's going very slowly. And it's very cold. So I end up helping her so that she doesn't feel cold, the food has to be fresh, she can't cook. So I do everything. Just like after I gave up, I still haven't managed to do all that cleaning [in her house],* (Dina)	Activities performed by the elderly person's family caregiver.
6	*So they support me too. Milito [...] The family gives me strength."* (Isabel)	Family support for caring for others.
7	*But we worry, right! I worry. I'm like: My God, what if I die? How is my father going to manage or him? [referring to o and sposo],* (Joshua)	Concern about dying due to dependence on the person being cared for, as well as fear of losing the other.
	So, I'm very scared, right, I was already attached to Auntie, and after I started looking after her, we're more attached every day, and if Auntie goes, I don't know what will become of me. [...] I'm just afraid that she'll go, but God is powerful, right? He doesn't give us a cross we can't bear. (Dina)	
8	*Yes. They help, but you know, they all have families, children, husbands and they live far away, so 'L...' [stepdaughter] is the one who helps the most, [but] she also has her [sens] children. I try to do what I can, only when I can't stand it, because [...] helps a lot, but she has children and a husband, she has her own life, right?* (Ruth)	The feeling of apprehension at being considered a burden to the family.
9	*So when I feel a lot of pain and I'm not well, I end up having to ask for help, I'm afraid of letting myself fall.* (Isabel)	
10	*God gives me strength, because I live in a jail without a*	Lifestyle changes related to the care

	wall [...]. (Ruth)	process.
11	*We overcome all the difficulties. And after it's over, we're like: how did I manage it? [...]. I don't think it's too much of a burden, because the moment we succeed, we have the capacity and strength to fight, right?* (Joshua)	Resilience in caring for others.
12	*Ah, my daughter, she's about 3 years old, and after that I only buy blood pressure medication. Sometimes my blood pressure gets too high, so I go back to the pharmacy, the girl looks at my blood pressure and that's it."* (Ruth)	Finding it difficult to take care of themselves.
13	*I go to church every Sunday. When I don't vote on Saturday, I vote on Sunday.* (Talita) *God helps me, because I have time for him. I watch Father Marcelo's Mass on TV and go back to church, because Father Marcelo's Mass is only good for those who can't afford to go to church. Now if you can go, you have to go there. Now there's a Sunday when you can't go, you can watch it on TV [no problem], it's not just early in the morning that there's Mass, there's the whole day, so it's valid, but you have to have time for God. Because, Our Lady, God helped me [...].* (Samuel)	Religious attendance as support and life support.
14	*Then I had to go to the pharmacy, ask the guy, and he even charged me twenty reais to come here and give her the injection, because she can't go without it, you know?* (Lia) *I know there's medicine at the clinic, but I don't have the money to get it and I end up having to buy it. If only someone who came to visit could bring it, it would help me a lot. We need it."* (Talita)	Care-seeking strategy/ Need for home care.
15	*The first thing I looked after was a paralyzed sister I had. She was born and ten years later she became paralyzed. Then I helped my mother [to] take care of her, I helped [to] take care of my father, who died thirteen years ago and, finally, I had to move to Cd to take care of my mother and my brother.* (Lia)	Previous experience cot o the process of caring for another person/ family member at home.
16	*I'm just afraid that I won't be able to hold on, because, as*	Weaknesses in exercising the role of

	I said, he's been getting worse, so I'm afraid that he'll fall, that he won't be able to hold on. (Ruth)	caregiver.
17	*[For example] cleaning the house: I started cleaning the house last Monday, in the bathroom; then, on Tuesday, I did the kitchen, you know? When it was Wednesday, I did her room, Friday I did the living room. It's like this, every day I do something, because I can't manage to do it all at once and I don't let myself either, you know?* (Lia)	Maintaining the home and environment in which the elderly person lives.
18	*[...] I can't afford it, I haven't retired. It's going to be very bad, but I have to say it, right? My daughter, who is from the federal tax office, made Sarah and me her dependents, because she was a very sick girl, she even had tuberculosis in her bones, and it cost a lot to cure it. In those days, tuberculosis was a big deal, right? And she had it, and because of that we couldn't pay and get our money. So she buys a health insurance plan [...] one that only treats inpatients, and it's very expensive, right? And the older we get...* (Adameire)	Financial dependence on another family member.
19	*It disgusts me to see [she starts to cry, com enormous suffering, o that moved me deeply: I wanted to cry together] her children don't care about her, it's all on my back, I suffer from seeing her suffer (there's a lot of sadness and anger at the lack of family support). [...] Look, it's a huge responsibility, right, because I'm on my own...* (Lia) *When I was in bed, I needed to go to the bathroom and I didn't have a way of getting there. I have a son who used to come here from time to time and help out, but not all the time, because he has his own house.* (Talita)	Little or no family support.
20	*It's changed... I don't go out much, I don't make friends, I don't have a social life, I have a life just for myself. I don't go back to my daughter's house, she lives here in Juiz de Fora.* (Adameire)	Leisure deficit.
21	*Everything like that, right? Her body was damaged, because she also worked, she also struggled to raise us, in the fields, right, because we lived in the fields. She*	Emotional burden of the elderly caregiver's role.

	fought, she cut sugar cane with me, with my father [she began to show a lot of emotion in her voice and her eyes were full of tears], she planted corn, beans, all this she did in the fields to help raise us. Then I hated her little body, and she sat there in that chair to	
	taking a bath with that deformed body, you know... (Lia)	
22	*And there's another thing I have: I'm very scared [crying]. This low wall, the way things are, nobody respects anyone, these things... [pause] I'm afraid of someone coming in with bad intentions, for example, there used to be his workshop here, when he stopped working I couldn't even walk inside it, there was so much iron all over the floor, now I go there to see if I've found a piece of iron.* (Adameire)	They feel unprotected and afraid of violence.
23	*And every time I get sick and I tell her I'm going to the doctor, wow, she freaks out, she won't let me. Eia can't be without me, I can't disappear... (listening to her mother looking for her in the living room)* (Lia)	Difficulty in moving away from the caregiver, due to the bond of trust established between them.
24	*Sometimes I go back to the yard to pray, sometimes I go back to the back, right? Because I don't want to cry near my daughter, right?"* (Lia) *So that's my struggle. There are days when I'm like this, sometimes I cry milito [her eyes filled with tears, and she smiled without motivation],* (Talita)	Expression of sadness.
25	*I don't get anything from anyone, nothing, only a few times from the health worker, who comes, but says that our area doesn't have a doctor. Even so, "N" [daughter who lives with the couple] got up early one day and went there [to the UAPS] to get the prescription for the tranquilizer we use, because without a prescription you can't buy medicine and, in this confusion, they lost my SUS card.* (Adameire) *The nurse, even last month [I asked her at this point to see if she knew the name of the nurse in charge of the area], [she answered] 'E', right? The one who gives*	Deficit in meeting the health needs of the elderly and dependent elderly caregivers.

	injections [actually the nursing technician]. Well, I used to give my mother the injection, every month, last month I called, I got tired of calling, asking, they didn't come to give my mother the injection. (Lia)	
26	*I take rheumatism medicine, I take blood pressure medicine, because I also have [high] blood pressure, [but] it's under control [...]* (Isabel) *I'm always at the doctor, trying to get better, sometimes I don't go because I'm lazy, but I do go, I have a cardiologist, an orthopedist, a gastroenterologist and a proctologist, [because] I have a problem with my hemorrhoids, I have diverticulitis, reflux [laughs], the things of age, right? But thank God, God has been giving me the strength to get as far as I have, because if he hadn't given me this strength, I would have given up.* (Talita)	Elderly people's knowledge of self-care.
27	*I'd really like to thank you for coming, for sitting me down. Wow, no one has ever stopped to listen to me. [Onero] apologize if I've said things that will hurt you. If if you want to come back, you'll always be very welcome.* (Dina) *Naie multo [to have a health professional who can listen], because sometimes we want someone to talk to, to explain our problems to someone who understands, and sometimes it happens that the people at home don't understand. Understand? Sometimes we want to talk...* (Talita)	The importance of active listening for the elderly.
28	*[...] In fact, things started to get complicated in 96, when she had a stroke, then, a year later, she had a seizure, and the doctor said that, after the stroke, she had to start taking phenobarbital [and], because she wasn't, she had a seizure. Now, after she's been with me, she's had two strokes, and now the doctor says she's starting Alzheimer's.* (Dina)	The aging process and the emergence of new pathologies.
29	*I needed serious treatment at the HU, but I was treated at*	Attending to the health needs of the

	the HU. Just yesterday we went to the rheumatologist, and when it was May last year, we discovered that she had osteoporosis. Until then we didn't know, she fell and fractured her pelvis, so she had to rest. When she had the plate removed, the doctor said: "You need to see a rheumatologist immediately, [because] she has osteoporosis." (Isabel)	dependent elderly.
30	*My daughter stays with me. For example, today I go out at 5 o'clock, [because] I do water aerobics. I do water aerobics three times a week.* (Isabel)	Preserved self-care of the elderly caregiver.
31	*I like to read the word. Not all the time, no, but there are a few psalms, Psalm 91 and Psalm 123, when I'm feeling that anguish, you know, that bad thing, I think that's normal, right?* (Dina) *I went to church every Sunday. When I haven't voted on Saturday, I've voted on Sunday. Or I go into my room and cry a lot, otherwise you can't stand it. I pray a lot, read the Bible. Then I leave the room feeling better. I go to mass every morning at Cançào Nova, because hearing the word of God helps a lot. Thanks be to God."* (Talita)	Religiosity as a strategy for relieving tension.
32	*I do everything com eia, so if eia goes to the doctor and [I] need it, Ciprove and consult me too. The people at the clinic are used to it."* (Dina)	He is accompanied by the ESF team.
33	*What happened next was that I began to notice some "strange things" [Long pause]. When I went to visit my mother, she was happier, but when it was time for her to leave, she wouldn't accept it, she insisted that I stay. So, every time I left, I left crying, you know? I told my sister, who lives in Uberlandia, that I was going to find a place to live with my mother, and she immediately agreed, saying: that's right, it'll be good for me."* (Dina)	Taking on the role of primary caregiver.
34	*Only [pause], with that, my family got upset with me, they thought, and one of my brothers even said, that I was only doing this out of interest in my mother's pension, or rather, her pensions, right?* (Dina)	Family conflict.

35	*I live there taking care of them, I go to the doctor, I get medicine at the gas station, but [for] myself nothing.* (Lia)	It prioritizes the needs of the person being cared for.
36	*Her house is very beautiful [referring to a daughter's house], but I didn't vote there either, because I can't, I don't have time.* (Adameire)	Lack of time.
37	*Look, we can't find any facilities. Especially [on] the part of the government, because there are no sidewalks for wheelchair users, there are no ramps. Then you get to a place that says it has a preferential, you'll stay there, you'll have to stay for 3, 4 hours.* (Gedeao)	Accessibility and lack of support from the public authorities straining the role of the caregiver.
38	*His money isn't even enough to buy medicine, it's a militant race for medicine.* (Adameire)	Economic aspects.
39	*When I got married, I was still Catholic, after I passed I know [pause] now I'm evangelical, but I always went [to church] and I took it seriously.* (Ruth)	Balance for daily coping, through personal search, regardless of religious affiliation.

5.4 AXIAL CODING

For each code previously identified, a related concept was generated in this second coding, in order to identify it through the data collected (TABLE 3).

TABLE 3 - Axial coding: forming concepts about the life context of the elderly family caregiver.

N.°	Codes	Conceptual Basis of Analysis
1	Growing old and becoming the main family caregiver.	They believe that they are responsible for caring for their family member as they get older, especially when they fall ill.
2	Spirituality/religiosity as strength and life support.	They place their hopes in a higher being. They believe that their life is governed by a Divine, superior force, which sustains them every day and keeps them alive and with the strength to go on forever.
3	Physical overload in the role of the elderly caregiver.	A state of physical exhaustion resulting from the routine of daily activities: activities or conditions related to the role of caregiver and others that represent an accumulation of tasks, which generate a physical impact on the caregiver and consequently compromise their health.

N.°	Codes	Conceptual Basis of Analysis
4	Compromised health of the elderly caregiver.	Reports of living with acute or chronic processes related or not to the process of caring for dependent elderly people who require permanent care, with professional monitoring or the use of medication.
5	Activities performed by the elderly person's family caregiver.	It represents the daily routine of caring for the dependent elderly relative, with the activities that, in the subjects' view, are the most strenuous.
6	Support received from family for self-care and caring for others.	Affirmations that when you have family support, everything is easier. Family support is very important in the process of taking care of others and helping them to take care of themselves.
7	Concern about dying due to dependence on the person being cared for, as well as fear of losing the other.	They are weakened by the feeling of losing their family member and, above all, they are afraid that they will be alone when they die. Or, on the contrary, they are afraid of dying and leaving the person they are caring for behind, and so questions arise, such as: what will become of them without me?
8	The feeling of apprehension at being considered a burden to the family.	They think they should solve their problems and carry out their activities as unaided as possible, because the other family members work and have families. So they believe that they should only resort to help when there's no way out.
N.°	Codes	Conceptual Basis of Analysis
9	Need for support from a secondary caregiver.	Activities and times when the main caregiver needs another family member/informal caregiver, taking turns and helping to reduce the burden.
10	Lifestyle changes related to the care process.	It shows the process that the person who, over time, becomes a caregiver goes through, which is when you have to change all or almost all of your life to meet the demands of the other person. Many believe that they "live in a jail without walls".
11	Resilience in caring for others.	Positive aspects or conditions that gave the caregiver a sense of well-being, the ability to cope with problems, to have new strength to overcome them, so that they could persevere and continue caring.

N.°	Codes	Conceptual Basis of Analysis
12	Finding it difficult to take care of themselves.	Signs of damage to the caregiver's self-care, as a result of the role played and in relation to hindering factors, such as lack of time and activities that bring physical and emotional overload.
13	Religious attendance as a support for coping with life.	They represent the manifestations of the elderly in relation to their faith and the importance of their frequent participation in religious services, as a form of support in coping with the misfortunes that arise during life.
14	Care-seeking strategy/ Need for home care.	The burden of care is passed on to the family, without adequate support from the state and with insipid home care, with sporadic actions by the health team.
15	Previous experience with the process of caring for another person/ family member at home.	They reported previous experience of caring for dependent individuals, which may have contributed positively to the current demand and provision of care for dependent family members.
16	Weaknesses in exercising the role of caregiver.	Caregivers report not being physically able to carry out the activity required by the person being cared for, often because they are also elderly and/or affected by pathology, or simply can't cope.
17	Maintenance of the house and environment	Report on the daily activities of caring for the environment in a concomitant way, generating overload.
18	Financial dependence on another family member.	When the caregiver is unable to meet all the expenses, usually because they don't have their own income for some reason.
19	Low or no family support.	For the elderly, this feeling seemed quite common. Reality expressed by the caregiver about their family reality: family members always have something more important to do, or even when other family members don't show up to help with the care demands and division of responsibilities.
		with the main caregiver.
N.°	Codes	Conceptual Basis of Analysis

20	Leisure deficit.	When we look at the abandonment of leisure activities in the routine of the caregiver, who reported having stopped doing activities such as traveling, parties, outings, etc.
21	Emotional burden of the elderly caregiver's role.	A state manifested by signs of stress, nervousness, anxiety, sadness and tension, associated with the activity of caring for dependent elderly people when compared to the lifestyle before becoming a caregiver.
22	They feel unprotected and afraid of violence.	They show a growing fear of being robbed, mugged and raped inside their own homes.
23	Difficulty in moving away from the person being cared for, due to the bond of trust that is created between them.	Feelings experienced by the caregiver, who shows difficulty in moving away from the dependent elderly person and insecurity in letting other people take over their care. And also because of the caregiver's reliance solely and exclusively on the family member who has taken over their care.
24	Expression of sadness.	Feelings experienced by the caregiver, such as discouragement and frustration, in relation to the attitude of family members and the health situation of the person they are caring for. This is often manifested by crying, insomnia, depression, nervousness, lack of appetite, among other things.
25	Deficit in meeting the health needs of the elderly and dependent elderly caregivers.	They report having a lot of difficulty getting care via the UAPS; they are not seen promptly, sometimes only the elderly person being cared for can get care and often they are left without the care they need.
26	Elderly people's knowledge of self-care.	Situation in which the elderly person demonstrates mastery of the care related to the treatment of their illness: care in the administration of medication, diet, application of insulin.
27	The importance of active listening for the elderly.	They show a need to talk, especially to be listened to. Generally, the caregiver is very overwhelmed by daily activities and is never listened to by anyone. And when this happens, it brings relief, it's a way of letting off steam.

N.°	Codes	Conceptual Basis of Analysis
28	The aging process and the emergence of new pathologies.	They understand the emergence of illnesses as a process that comes with aging, leading to an increase in the caregiver's burden in the process of caring for others.
29	Attention to the health needs of the dependent elderly.	This includes the search for care in the private network, outpatient care, emergency services and hospital care.
N.°	Codes	Conceptual Basis of Analysis
30	Preserved self-care of the elderly caregiver.	Maintaining the caregiver's ability to meet self-care needs.
31	Religiosity as a strategy for relieving tension.	Activities they carry out: either in the pursuit of religion, through frequent participation, when they say their prayers in their own homes, or even when they watch religious programs on TV or listen to them on the radio, as a way of relieving the burden of everyday life.
32	Follow-up by the ESF team.	From the point of view of the elderly, the presence of a health professional can make their day-to-day lives easier, as it helps them learn activities and how to deal with pathology; it also serves as a source of information. In addition to better care for the person being cared for.
33	Taking on the role of primary caregiver.	Sometimes it's necessary to take on the role of caregiver in the place of the other family member who, until then, had been fulfilling the role, especially when it's clear that the loved one is in need, is in a precarious hygiene situation or even when, for some reason, even health reasons, the other person is no longer able to fulfill this role.
34	Family conflict.	It happens when a family member takes on the responsibility of caring for the dependent elderly person. Or even when one or more family members do not accept the role played by the caregiver. It also indicates any situation in which the caregiver feels vulnerable about the role or actions of their family members.
35	It prioritizes the needs of the person being cared for.	Even though there are two elderly people involved, the caregiver makes a point of prioritizing, at all times, the

N.°	Codes	Conceptual Basis of Analysis
		care needs of the person being cared for (be it hygiene, health, food and so on), often giving up self-care.
36	Lack of time.	This factor has been identified as responsible for the difficulty in meeting the caregiver's self-care needs and relieving tension, as well as causing physical and emotional overload.
37	Accessibility and low public support.	Lack of roads to facilitate access for wheelchair users, such as ramps and bus stops. In the opinion of the caregivers, these are simple things that would make their job easier.
N.°	**Codes**	**Conceptual Basis of Analysis**
38	Economic aspects.	Situations in which the caregiver reported difficulties, such as increased costs and compromised health.
		family budget, without anyone to turn to.
39	Balance for daily coping, through personal search, regardless of religious affiliation.	The change of religious affiliation is due to a family link or the search for strength to face life.

5.5 SELECTIVE CODING

In this phase, the four categories were formed and related to their subcategories, in an attempt to generate more concise and complete explanations of the phenomenon studied "The life of the elderly and the process of caring for an elderly family member at home." (TABLE 4).

TABLE 4 - The life of the elderly and the process of caring for an elderly relative at home.

CATEGORY1 - GROWING OLD AND BECOMING A FAMILY CAREGIVER

SUBCATEGORY 1	The process of caring for others in everyday life.	Growing old and becoming the main family caregiver.
		Taking on the role of primary caregiver.
		Previous experience with the process of caring for another person/family member at home.
		Prioritizing the needs of the person being cared for.

		Compromised health of the elderly caregiver.
		Lifestyle changes related to the care process.
SUBCATEGORY 2	Being a family caregiver and its implications for health and self-care.	Activities performed by the elderly family caregiver.
		Weaknesses in exercising the role of caregiver.
		Maintaining the home and the environment in which the elderly person lives.
		Leisure deficit.
		Lack of time.
		Difficulty in moving away from the person being cared for, due to the bond of trust that is created between them.

CATEGORY 2 - FAMILY SUPPORT		
SUBCATEGORY 1	Family support positively influencing the process of caring for others.	Support received from family to care for others and self-care.
		Preserved self-care of the elderly caregiver.
		Need for support from a secondary caregiver
SUBCATEGORY 2	The absence of family support negatively influences the care of others and the health of the caregiver.	Low or no family support.
		Feeling unprotected and afraid of violence.
		Economic aspects.
		Financial dependence on another family member.
		A sense of apprehension at being

		considered a burden to the family.
		Family conflict.
		Difficulty with self-care.
		Expression of sadness.
		Physical overload in the role of the elderly caregiver.
		Emotional burden of the elderly caregiver's role.

CATEGORY 3 - THE SPIRITUAL DIMENSION INFLUENCING THE LIFE AND CARE PROCESS OF THE CENTRAL ELDERLY FAMILY CAREGIVER

SUBCATEGORY 1	Spirituality/Religio sity: a foundation for the life of the elderly.	Spirituality/religiosity as strength and life support.
		Balance for daily coping, through personal search, regardless of religious affiliation.
		Religious attendance as a support for coping with life.
		Religiosity as a strategy for relieving tension.
CATEGORY 2	The spiritual dimension: strength and motivation to continue caring for others.	Concern about dying, due to dependence on the person being cared for, as well as fear of losing the other.
		Resilience in caring for others.

CATEGORY 4 - THE Elderly CAREGIVER WHO CARES DAILY FOR AN ELDERLY PERSON IN THE HOME AND THE HEALTH TEAM .

SUBCATEGORY I	Health services and the need for home care	The aging process and the emergence of new pathologies.
		Deficit in meeting the health needs of the elderly and dependent elderly caregivers.
		Strategies for seeking care/ Need for

		home care .
		Attention to the health needs of the dependent elderly.
		Accessibility and low public support.
SUBCATEGORY 2	Contributions of the health team to the comprehensive care of the elderly caregiver-elderly family member binomial.	The importance of active listening for the elderly.
		Accompanied by the ESF team.
		Elderly people's knowledge of self-care.

Based on the methodological framework used to analyze the material collected, four categories related to the object of the study emerged. The category "The spiritual dimension influencing the life and care process of the elderly family caregiver" stands out as the central category of the study, compared to the other three categories, which are nevertheless related to each other (DIAGRAM 1).

This category was considered by us to be the central category, as it has the capacity to bring together the other categories to form an explanatory whole. The study focused on issues of spirituality/religiosity from the very first interview, based on the data collected, without the researcher making any inference in this regard. It should be noted that the interviews did not initially focus on this issue of religiosity/spirituality, but rather on the self-care of the elderly caregiver, which was the initial assumption for the study. People at this stage of life have shown themselves to be spiritual and have an individualized view of the meaning of life. An experienced view, acquired through their experiences, which have not always been the easiest. Today, despite all their experiences as family carers of a person who depends on them, they are grateful and look to the transcendent for the strength to continue living and caring, vehemently guaranteeing that all things are only possible with the help of a higher being who, for them, is God.

DIAGRAM 1 - Relationship between the categories of the study, highlighting the central category.

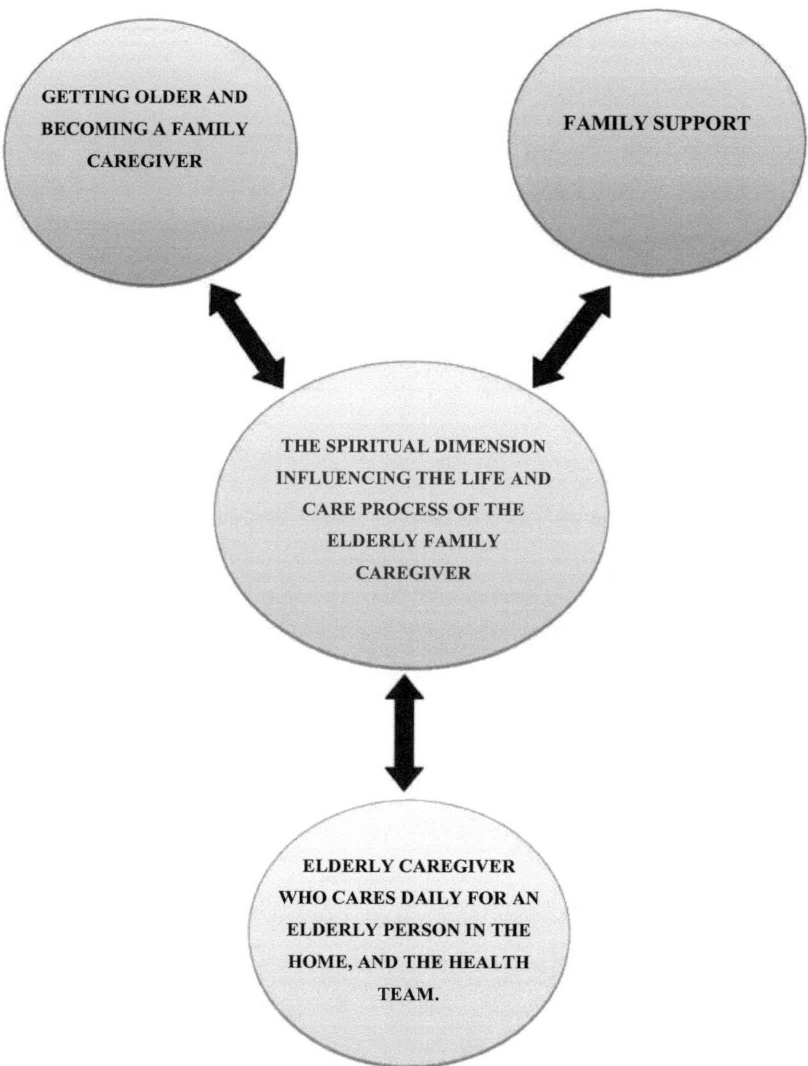

The following is an analysis and discussion of the four categories established in the study, with their related subcategories.

5.6 -THE SPIRITUAL DIMENSION INFLUENCING THE LIFE AND CARE PROCESS OF THE ELDERLY FAMILY CAREGIVER (CENTRAL CATEGORY)

Based on the data found in this study and in line with the scientific literature, it can be understood that, as the years go by, that is, during the ageing process, people tend to re-signify the meaning of life, from perspectives such as: redefining the meaning of relationships; changes in point of view; and a new perception of the speed of time between past, present and future, where the past is recalled in a way that has never been experienced before. In this phase of life, the person is searching for wisdom, is less self-centered and begins to have an intense relationship with the spiritual dimension, through the personal search for something greater and that brings strength to face life's adversities. Below is an excerpt from one of her last interviews:

My strength comes from God, the day I don't say my prayers, I'm missing something, it's the faith I have in God, regardless of family or anything else, what drives me is the faith I have in God. It's always in my life, always at his discretion. (Samuel)

The experience of searching for the sacred generates a profound transformation in the being and makes it integrated with itself and the world, giving life a new meaning. An endless human search for meaning and personal significance. According to Müller (2004, p. 31): "when I can reach the innermost part of myself, I am in contact with the world of the sacred (...)".

It was understood in this study, according to the interviewees, that with the support of family members, the process of caring for others becomes lighter; however, without their spiritual needs being met, there is a weakening of their empowerment, because in religion they find the strength to face life and care for others, as well as their own awareness of growing old. The essence of religiosity is to sustain and develop the individual's relationship with the sacred. Its purpose is to give meaning to life. In this way, it can provide support for the individual to transcend suffering, loss and the perception of death (GOLDSTEIN & SOMMERHALDER, 2002). Corroborating the above, take a look at the following speech by a 90-year-old research participant, who currently looks after her daughter and husband, both elderly, and effectively has minimal family support:

I don't take a drop of water in the morning until I thank God, I thank him for my life, the lives of my children, my husband, the house is in pieces, but it's mine, I thank him for everything. I believe that God is the one who gives strength, everyone, everything we go through is by his will, if we fail to understand or desire his presence with us, we have no life, our life is the divine light, it's God's strength. (Adameire)

In this elderly woman's account, we can see that she goes about her daily life with a view to what is really called integral care, which is being with the other, even with the frailties that come with the ageing process. Health professionals, especially ESF nurses, should pay attention to their public in order to access the spiritual dimension as a way of providing individual, quality care.

Referring to spirituality in primary health care, Smeke (2006) proposes that, in everyday care, whether through consultations, in groups or at home, professionals are often faced with an intricate web of needs, complaints and pains, which blend together, entangling and going beyond the limits of the illness. During this period, suffering visibly goes beyond the organic relationship and "if we really want to help, we must step out of our professional role and put our human side into action" (SMEKE, 2006, p. 298). When the professional comes into contact with the dimension that goes beyond the psychosomatic space of the person being cared for, and through the act of welcoming, of qualified listening, it sparks understanding, hope and the relief of pain and suffering.

One issue observed during the interviews, in the participants' speeches, were some of the expressions used by the elderly people which, due to the intonation of their voices and the way they were said, were not just a simple everyday expression, but were intended to express faith and devotion. They often use the expressions "Se Deus quiser" and "Graças a Deus", as can be seen below:

Like my mother, thank God, my mother doesn't have any problems, because with age they don't like taking a bath, she loves taking a bath, she loves dyeing her hair, putting on make-up, she loves it. That's very good [...] everything's fine with me, right?

Sometimes we feel sad for no reason. As human beings, every day you wake up in a different way. But it's not because of what I do on a daily basis, it's because it's human, but then I start singing, I find someone to smile a bit, because smiling is good for you, and on we go, thanks be to God. (Gedeao)

So that day [referring to church duties], he doesn't leave until I arrive because I have to get strength from God, so that I have the strength to sort everything out at home. [...] So that's it, God helps me! I can handle it, thank God, and if God wants me to, for as long as they need me to (Joshua).

In his study on *Religiosity and health: patients' experiences and professionals' perceptions*, Freitas (2014) emphasizes the expressions Brazilians often hear when asked about their health condition. These include: "Everything's fine, thank God!" or "I'm going to get better, God willing!". These translate into a pattern of how important religiosity is in the lives of these people and how much they themselves relate it to their physical, mental or spiritual well-being (FREITAS, 2014).

The author also questions whether health professionals recognize the importance of these expressions in the context of the various health services in our country. Is there any room in the scientific rationality that regulates professional training for listening to the religious faith that moves their patients? Or should these statements be considered mere reflections of naive perspectives that have nothing to do with the scientific knowledge that underpins their clinical practices?

DIAGRAM 2 - The spiritual dimension influencing the care process of an elderly family caregiver - central category

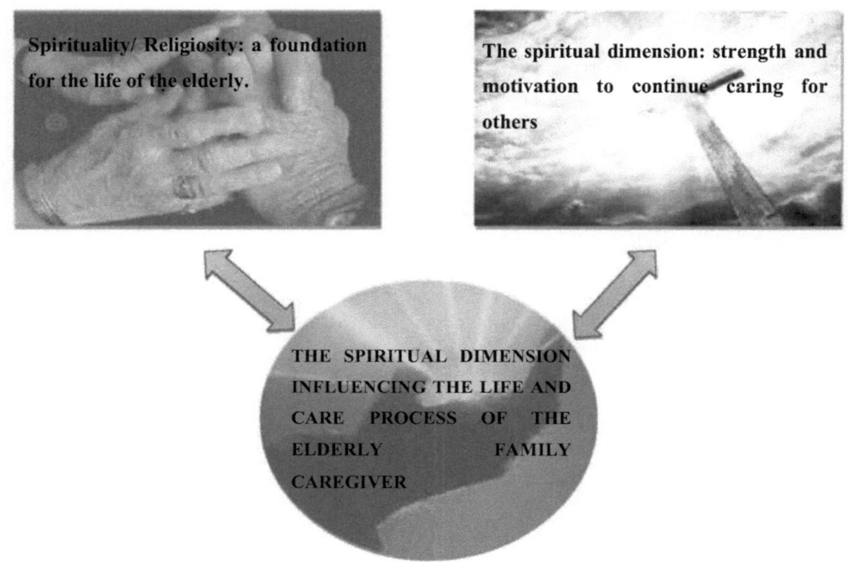

5.6.1 Spirituality/Religiosity: the foundation of life for the elderly

There is a consensus in the literature that, in the ageing phase, religiosity plays a central role in the lives of the elderly. They use religion to cope better with their difficulties, illnesses and even death (DALGALARRONDO, 2008). The study by Manning (2013) suggests that spirituality is important for a respectable portion of the elderly population and acts as a factor in promoting healthy ageing. It also highlights that participants use their spirituality as a tool to promote and maintain resilience over the years in their lives (MANNING, 2013).

Brazil is considered to be a religious country, and Brazilians have shown that they hold to some form of belief, although over the years there has been a loss of Catholic hegemony. According to the interpretation of the last IBGE census, in 2010, a new phase is emerging, which shows an increase in the number of adherents to other faiths, including Protestant, Spiritualist and others. However, the census showed that only 8% of the total population declared themselves to be "without religion", which includes the categories: without religion, atheist and agnostic (those who declared an undetermined/ ill-defined religion or declared multiple religions). It can also be seen that atheists make up only 0.3% of the population and agnostics less than 0.1%. It should be noted that approximately 4.3% of people aged 60 or over declared themselves to be "without religion", which includes the same questions mentioned above (IBGE, 2012).

For the authors, the person gives religion their main motivation (STROPPA; MOREIRA-ALMEIDA, 2008). Religiosity is not just a feeling of self-perception on the part of the individual, as it encompasses an action of affirmation or denial in relation to concrete issues that transform people's personalities, being inseparable elements (VALLE 2002).

So, we will start from the following premise: to what extent is religion part of the life of an elderly person? Based on the participants' accounts, it is clear that religiosity is of significant importance in their lives, as they state that:

Religion is important for each and every human being, since "FAITH" [I emphasize when talking about faith] makes us believe in everything we want and that can be achieved. (Samuel)

Faith removes mountains. You have to believe, have faith, and God gives us intuition, gives us direction [in the sense of wisdom for the decision to be taken]. (Gedeao)

And the reason for this seems to be simple: believing that there is a 'supreme force', something that can't be seen, but can be imagined, and having faith ends up becoming a respite to overcome the obstacles and burdens - many of them heavy - that life throws at you along the way.

This is reflected in their daily lives, in their ability to express multiple forms of religious beliefs, which are a fundamental part of their lives. This is a common tradition in Brazilian culture and the analysis of the reports made it possible to identify the manifestations of the elderly in relation to what they seek and believe in, emerging the code: **Spirituality/Religiosity as strength and life support,** which they point to as the main form of support for their empowerment and daily coping with the illness and the process of caring for others, even when they have no other form of support in caring for their dependent loved one.

He got very bad, he was hospitalized [pause] for many months and was practically disillusioned. When the doctor saw him walking again, he said it was a miracle [pause]. From then on, I started taking care of him and thank God I'm still taking care of him today. And God has been giving me strength [...] some people still ask me how can you stand it? God gave me this cross to carry. The important thing is faith. [pause] It's not easy [laughs], but God gives me strength. [...] But I'll carry on as long as God gives me life and health. (Ruth)

It's God's, it's God, right, because if I didn't have the faith I have in God, I don't think I'd be here anymore [he suggested by the tone of his voice that he would have done something] [short pause]. I even asked God, if it's a sin, I asked God, for God to take her, because I don't understand why she's suffering so much, does she have so much sin? Isn't it? I asked God to take her, but don't let her suffer any more, because I can't bear to see her suffer any more.

But that's the strength we have to draw on. It's in God, I look to God, I look to Him to strengthen me every day. When I get up every morning, I say: Thank you very much for the night, and thank you for another day that is beginning. Every day I say thank you, He gives me strength and the love I feel for my husband. Love gives us incredible strength. And this love goes back many years, it's very beautiful, our love story is very beautiful, if he were still writing it, it would be a beautiful book, a novel, but God gives me strength. [brief pause]. Yes, with God I can overcome anything, I say to him, come on my son, strengthen your legs, with God we can do it, with family or without family we can overcome anything. (Eunice)

While they seek support from a metaphysical force, the participants also attribute to the divine the strength to persevere and continue along their path, growing old and caring for one or more elderly people at home. From the participants' statements, we can see the presence of religious-spiritual *coping* which, according to Panzini and Bandeira (2005), are the strategies of religiosity and spirituality employed to deal with difficult life circumstances.

In a study carried out, religious *coping* showed a positive relationship with quality of life and better levels of physical health. It showed a positive relationship with positive changes in subjective health perception, cognitive functioning and general physical state. In terms of spiritual health, there was a positive relationship with the feeling of connection to God, the feeling of closeness to others and feelings of spiritual growth (PARGAMENT et al., 2003, PARGAMENT; ANO, 2004).

Because we have God with us [laughs], because with God, we have the strength for everything, right? [short pause] We feel victorious because we made it. (Joshua)

It's a lot of responsibility, but I thank God every morning because God has given me grace and strength. Sometimes when I think I'm not going to make it, God renews me [pause, thoughtful] So these are things that make us sad, there are days when we want to cry, but then God says to me: son, I'm giving you strength, I'm giving you strength, go ahead. So that's what's holding me up, holding me up and I'm going, I'm walking and God has given me this Grace. [...] I just have to thank God for the strength he gives me. Gedeao

Coping strategies based on religiosity include the use of religion, spirituality or faith to deal with anxiety, stress and the negative consequences generated by the experience of everyday problems (PANZINI; BANDEIRA, 2005, 2007).

Based on the analysis of the data and according to the Religious-Spiritual *Coping* Scale (CRE Scale), which has been translated, adapted and validated in terms of construct, criteria and content of the Religious-Spiritual *Coping* Scale (PANZINI, 2004), based on the North American RCOPE scale (PARGAMENT; KOENIG; PEREZ, 2000), Table 5 below highlights the positive *coping* strategies used by the caregivers participating in this study in their daily lives.

TABLE 5 - *Coping* strategies commonly used by the caregivers participating in the study.

Factors	Strategy used
Changes in yourself and/or your life	*They just* think it's important to ask for forgiveness and to be forgiven for their mistakes.
Actions in search of spiritual help	S Attending religious/spiritual services.
Helping others	S Trying to provide spiritual comfort to other people. S Praying for the well-being of others. S Offering spiritual support to others.
Positive attitude towards God	S Seek God's love and protection. They believe that God is always with them. S Look to God for strength, support and guidance. Just pray to God that everything will be all right. He feels that God is working on his behalf. S Establishes a greater connection with God.
Actions in search of institutional aid	S Listening to and/or singing religious songs. S Performing spiritual acts or rites (any action specifically
	related to their belief: sign of the cross, confession, praying the rosary, fasting, purification rituals, quoting proverbs, chanting mantras, psychography, etc.) S Taking part in religious or spiritual practices, activities or festivities. S Going to a religious temple. S Keep a place of prayer at home.

	S Seeking spiritual support from the leaders of my religious community.
	S Seek the house of God.
Personal search for spiritual knowledge	S Seek help from the holy books (Bible and others).
	S Seeking help or comfort in religious literature.
	S Watching religious or spiritual programs or films.
	S Reading books on spiritual/religious teachings to understand and deal with adversity.

From the analysis of the data obtained in this study, it was identified that the participants show flexibility in changing their religious beliefs, with the code emerging: **Balance for daily coping, through personal search, regardless of their religious affiliation**. Take a look at the participants' statements:

When I got married I was still Catholic, after I passed [pause] although when I was Catholic I always liked practicing, because there are people who take it as a joke, you know, one hour they go and another they don't, just like Catholics, one hour they go well and another hour they don't. I've always dedicated myself, I've always liked going to Mass. I've always dedicated myself, I've always liked going to Mass. I've always been dedicated." (Ruth)

I stay, [...]. Six o'clock this morning I was watching the pastor on the Record network. [...] That's what I do every morning, when I'm watching the pastor, he's not even from the Catholic church, he's from the evangelical church, you know? Which I really like listening to, because God is one, right, whatever church you go to, God is there, it's the same, it's not, nothing changes. (Lia)

I'm actually Catholic, but I haven't been to church for a long time. Actually, [laughs awkwardly] lately I've been going to the evangelical church, because my brother, you know, mom doesn't answer much for her, and he took her to his church and baptized her, so because of her I started going, but really, I don't think it matters, right? (Dina)

According to Moreira-Almeida (2010), religiosity has been recognized as an important source of support among people in learning to cope with stressful circumstances and it is believed that there is a positive association between religiosity and improved quality of life and good mental health.

Much has been discussed around the terms used, in reality, the way individuals experience their spiritual experience, which can happen through religiosity. For Allport (1950), mental health is positively related to the experience of intrinsic religiosity. The author justifies this statement by the greater awareness and resistance to external pressures displayed by the individual who experiences this type of religious practice and is thus able to distance themselves from the emotional effects of external pressures.

It can be seen from the reports that the interviewees are looking for internalized feelings to give meaning to their existence and empowerment for their daily work:

Only God, you have to have a lot of faith, ask him for protection. [pause] [...] Girl, I don't know where this strength comes from, you know, where the strength doesn't come from, but I know that God is helping me, he's helping me because I think it's only him to give us the strength, to keep living, right, because life is very difficult, it's everything, everything for me today is difficult, but then as I always ask God, I ask him for protection, I ask him for help, for the light to be able to enlighten me, especially to finish taking care of my mother. (Lia)

I like to read the word, not all the time, but there are some psalms, like Psalm 91 and Psalm 123, when I'm feeling that anguish, you know, that bad thing, I think that's normal, right? Everyone feels it, so I ask God, because he's the greatest force, right? It's where we get the strength to go on with our lives, and I believe that he doesn't abandon us, he doesn't forsake us, he's always with us [he showed a lot of peace and wisdom when he spoke, a lot of sincerity in his tone]. There are no different Gods, only one, and not one for each church. (Dina)

According to the authors, people with high levels of intrinsic religiosity find greater meaning in life through religiosity/spirituality, as they often internalize the basic principles of their beliefs, which will determine the meaning of their existence (KOENIG; BÜSSING, 2010).

According to Koenig and Büssing (2010), organizational religiosity is the individual's religious participation in churches, temples, synagogues, and can be in events such as: masses, services, prayer groups, scripture study groups, religious meetings and others involving the topic. Religious attendance is considered to be the constancy with which an individual attends a religious service (ASSOCIATION OF RELIGION DATA ARCHIVES, 1998).

In order to represent the manifestations that the elderly reveal in relation to their faith and the importance of their frequent participation in religious services, as a form of support in coping with the misfortunes that arise during life, the code emerged: **religious attendance as support for coping with life.**

I take part in church things, one day a week I take communion to the sick. [...] It's praying, going to church, looking for meetings, because for me to go to church, there's nothing to hold me back, sometimes he says: I'm going to lie down. I say you're going to lie down and I'm going to pray, because we have a rosary there every Wednesday, on Thursdays and Tuesdays it's in church, I'm Catholic, the girls invite me, because I'm also in the baptism ministry, so the meeting after six o'clock is enough for me to go. A prayer helps a lot. Because we get closer, there talking to God, right! And we say our prayers. So that day [referring to church duties], he doesn't leave until I get there because I have to get strength from God, so that I have the strength to sort everything out at home. [...] So that's it, God helps me! I can handle it, thank God, and if God wants me to, for as long as they need me to (Joshua).

Now we have to have faith in God. I'm Catholic, but someone with another religion has his own methods. Sometimes she's sick, she likes to sleep with the fan on, it's bad for me, it dries out my nose, I've had adenoid surgery. Then I start praying and by the time I've finished, she's asleep. This is a blessing that God helps me with, because I have time for him. I watch Father Marcelo's mass on TV and I go to church every week, because Father Marcelo's mass is only for those who can't afford to go to church, now if you can afford to go to church, you have to go there. (Samuel)

I go to church every Sunday, when I don't go on Saturday, I go on Sunday. (Talita)

It can be understood from the data presented so far that the process of caring for another elderly person is not an easy task, especially when the caregiver is also elderly. This is linked to the fact that few caregivers have any kind of support from their families. Faced with the challenges that arise on a daily basis, they turn to **religion as a strategy for relieving tension**.

First of all, I can't go without going to Mass. And I love going to the mall, I love shopping, I may not have the money to buy, but I love the windows, I love shopping. So I'm not doing that much, but sometimes I go to the doctor's, then [pause] I go to the mall a bit, but you know? I don't do it every day, you know, so as not to make her feel too much, right? She's not as comfortable as she is with me, when she's with my little girl. (Isabel)

And during the time that he sometimes goes out [referring to her husband], during the day, because I don't really like television, I really like music. I turn on the radio quietly, listening to praise music. (Joshua)

I believe that religion helps us a lot, because we look for it." (Ruth)

Koenig, MCCullough and Larson (2001) state that religious participation can help relieve depressive symptoms, mainly thanks to the psychological resources provided by various types of religious institution. Regardless of creed, religious experience can lead to consequences in the way a person lives, being constantly associated with greater detachment from things, as well as the acquisition of a sense of fraternity and commitment to solving human problems, in addition to a deeper feeling of joy (BAUNGART; AMATUZZI 2007).

5.6.2 The spiritual dimension: strength and motivation to keep laughing at others

As the years go by, the person becomes more reflective, tends to rethink their life, tracing its entire trajectory, arriving at the present day and evaluating how it was and how it will be from then on. Thus, the study highlighted the issue of **concern about dying due to dependence on**

being cared for, as well as the fear of losing others. The participants reported being afraid of their own death, due to their role as a caregiver and their dependence on others and, on the other hand, the fear of losing the person closest to them, with whom they share their days and nights in a relationship of intimacy and reciprocity. They showed a lot of emotion when referring to death, and were firm in their search for a supreme being who protects them, gives them strength and never abandons them:

So, I'm very scared, right, I was already attached to her, and after I started looking after her, we're more attached every day, and if she goes, I don't know what will become of me. [...] I'm just scared that she'll go, but God is powerful, right? He doesn't give us a cross we can't bear. (Dina)

And his fear is [pause]. I say: I want to go after him, I say: I'm going to suffer a lot, but if he stays here alone he'll suffer a lot more. So I don't want him to suffer. All those reports of old people in nursing homes on television, all of them mistreated, he cried, I don't want to. I'd say to him: as long as I'm alive and healthy, you're not going to any nursing home, you're not going, and I have faith in God that you'll go before me, I'd say to him. Because then you won't suffer." (Eunice)

According to Koenig, MCCullough and Larson (2001), the anxiety caused by the fear of death tends to decrease as the elderly become more spiritual. And so, during consultations with the elderly, caring for them using religiosity also means building a social support network in practice, pointing to the possibility of coping with health and illness problems (LINDOLPHO; SA; ROBERS, 2009).

Based on the understanding of resilience as the individual's ability to adapt and transform situations of risk, stress and vulnerability into potential, a correlation is made with the caregivers in this study who, even in the face of adversity, find positive aspects or conditions that provide a sense of well-being, so that they can persevere and continue caring. It was possible to identify in the interviewees' reports that the care relationship is surrounded by a variety of feelings which directly reflect the daily lives of the caregivers, whether through difficulties and suffering or through overcoming and developing **resilience in caring for others:**

But thank God [...] We overcome all the difficulties. And after it's over, we're like, how did I manage it [pause]. I don't think it's too much of a burden, because the moment we succeed, we have the ability and the strength to fight, right?

To say that it's gratifying isn't right, because seeing the person you love immobilized, but for the love that God has had for us, has blessed us with, I'm happy, because I have to thank God for always giving me this strength, this immensity, this love that I have, not only for her, because she's my wife, but for all the people around me, and who need me for something, I'm always ready to do whatever I can. (Gedeao)

For Walsh (2005), resilience is "the ability to be reborn from adversity stronger and with more resources" (p. 4). And he clarifies that this: "is an active method of resistance, restructuring and growth in response to crisis and challenge", when he refers to a "rebirth". The author highlights the process of transformation that takes place as a result of facing adversity, and also stresses that resilience is built through adversity, as a result of people's encounters with it. She also emphasizes that life's crises and difficulties can bring out the best in human beings, as long as the challenges are faced (WALSH, 2005).

Over the years, man's withdrawal from his spiritual quest was directly reflected in nursing care, a profession which, in its historical context, was associated with religious precepts (LINDOLPHO; SA; ROBERS, 2009). Still, according to the authors, Florence managed to structure nursing as a professional practice, whose inspiration and basis were interspersed with religiosity, but which established the scientific principles that guided her work, based on statistics, thus establishing the breaking of a paradigm (LINDOLPHO; SA; ROBERS, 2009).

During nursing consultations at home, nurses should be concerned with caring for elderly caregivers and their families, taking into account their bio-psycho-spiritual needs. The whole person must be considered; a person cannot be fragmented; it is important that they are seen in an integral way, with a view to valuing the positive feelings expressed by caregivers during their daily care.

Health professionals must remain alert to the needs related to the spiritual dimension of the person and be sensitized to this aspect in the search for health care based on a humanistic view of the person. It is therefore important to use spirituality as an auxiliary element in the process of health care for the elderly, given that spirituality is heightened at this stage of life.

In the course of this new experience for the caregivers and following their care routines, it was observed that, despite the numerous difficulties faced, especially in the initial phase of building the role of caregiver, in which fear, insecurity and inexperience are still frequent, over time, family members move to adapt to their new living conditions and try to overcome these obstacles. Empowerment and security to carry out care are then the phase in which the elderly family caregiver, faced with their uninterrupted care experiences, solidifies an experience and gradually begins to adapt to the needs of care. In addition to adapting to care routines, they create strategies for better care, with effectiveness and safety, based on a spiritual vision that conditions them to continue caring, with safety and autonomy. From the moment they acquire autonomy, possibilities arise for better coping, in all senses: bio-psycho-social and spiritual. Therefore, the work of professional nurses with a view to continuing health education can shorten the process of adaptation and, consequently, the elderly person will gain more time for themselves.

Look, I feel safe, I don't know because every day I feel, I don't know, I'm being renewed, driven by a greater force that keeps me on my feet. Then there are days when [quick pause] I wake up at 5:30, 6 o'clock, then my body isn't asking for it, my body doesn't want to get up, but then I get angry with it, you're not the boss of me, I'm the boss of you. So you won't beat me, because if I get up late, I'll delay her medication. Gedeao

During the interviews, it was clear from the words of each caregiver that their needs are not limited to objective issues, but permeate the field of subjectivity and spirituality. Therefore, there are circumstances experienced by elderly caregivers that need to be addressed by health professionals in the care provided, tending to constitute a configuration for the balance of their being. In this way, the management of spirituality proves to be effective, especially in the care of the elderly.

In view of the historical context of spirituality throughout human history, we believe that there is a strong need to implement it in health care, as a way of valuing the human being, based on the spiritual dimension; as well as comprehensive care for the being, with a focus on the spirituality they bring as a way of valuing each person's life story. Starting with respect and appreciation, new paths will emerge for assistance in the health-disease process. To do this, professionals will have to give new meaning to their practice, awakening to a new way of looking at the patient/user. It is believed that professionals have the capacity to rescue subjectivity and the integration of the entire human dimension.

5.7 - GROWING OLD AND BECOMING A FAMILY CAREGIVER

Until recently, aging was considered something distant and, when it was reached, it was perceived as synonymous with illness. Therefore, if a person reached the age of 60-70, from then on, staying alive, whatever the conditions, was considered a profit. Today, we are experiencing an accelerated ageing process and the scientific community is looking for ways to ensure that this phase is lived in an active and healthy way. And in this context, one figure becomes crucial: the family caregiver. The first category of the study helps us to understand the definition of the ageing process and the life process, which leads the elderly to become the main carer for their elderly family member. Generally, this happens because of chronic conditions, degenerative processes and health sequelae, compromising the capacity for self-care, as well as triggering the process of becoming dependent, so that they can no longer perform the basic and/or instrumental activities of daily living.

From then on, family structures need to be arranged, because in most cases a single member is chosen, either by obligation or by the person's own choice. This is when the family member becomes the main caregiver. In this particular study, the caregiver is elderly and has become a caregiver because he or she considers him or herself responsible for the life of the person they care for, either through family ties or affection.

This category is approached through two subcategories: the process of caring for others in everyday life and being a family caregiver and its implications for health and self-care, which brings up the stages of aging itself and the daily process of caring for a dependent elderly family member.

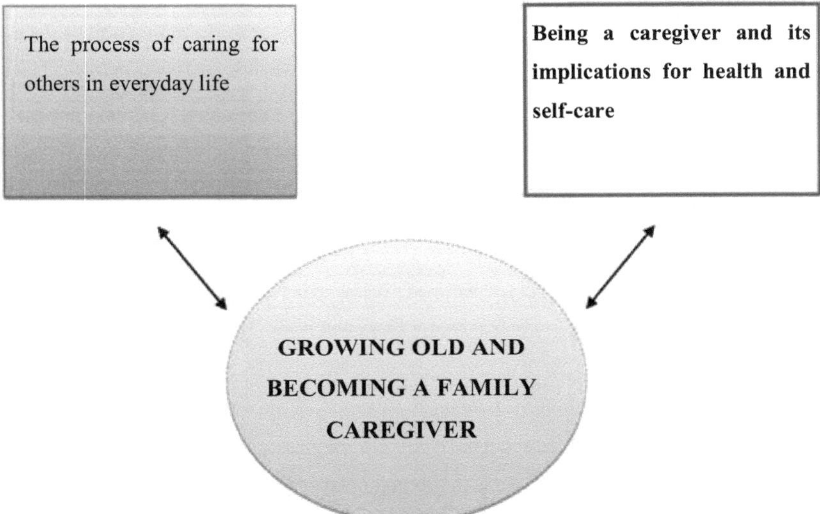

5.7.1 The process of caring for others in everyday life

With the process of population aging, taking on the task of family caregiver has become a common event in society. In this process, the role of caregiver has become that of the elderly person, even if they don't have adequate preparation, knowledge or support to perform this function.

From the observations and interviews carried out with elderly caregivers in their homes, it was possible to gain a better understanding of how the process of **growing old and becoming the main family caregiver takes place.** It emerged that the process of elderly dependency begins with the gradual loss of the ability to carry out basic activities of daily living, usually as a result of disabilities arising from health problems. The 11 (remembering that one elderly woman cares for her daughter and husband, both elderly) elderly people cared for by the family member showed a high degree of dependence in basic activities, requiring the presence of a caregiver to attend to or help with their self-care needs. In particular, they were unable to bathe, dress, feed themselves, walk and have continence. It can be seen that the onset of the caregiver role does not always happen abruptly, but progressively, as the elderly lose their ability to take care of themselves. This can be understood from the following statements:

I started looking after her from then on. It's been four years, and in those four years, we moved away, separated from her daughter because we couldn't live together. So we moved out on our own, and I started taking care of her. (Gedeao)

It was very difficult, he had a stroke in 2000 and his whole left side was paralyzed [...], then there were no sequelae, none of that, then he started to get weak in the leg, he got weak, he would sit on the pot, he couldn't get up. Then, in 2007, about seven years later, he started to lose his legs. (Eunice)

He had three strokes, the first was 32 years old and left him three years old, and left him practically unable to walk, he was 48 at the time, but with a lot of treatment he managed to recover his movements. Then, in 1999, he got prostate cancer and had radical surgery to remove everything. Then he had toxoplasmosis, and I was always looking after him, because from the time he had the stroke, he couldn't think of anything else to do. Then, in 2008, he had another stroke, this one he had, because the first one left him unable to walk, but he recovered because of his age, [he was] 48. The 2008 stroke left him unable to walk, and to this day he's on a walker, in a wheelchair, with a cane, he walks by leaning on walls. (Talita)

On the other hand, for some elderly people, the caregiving process begins after an abrupt event, such as a stroke that leaves sequelae or due to various causes and even advanced age does not allow for a satisfactory recovery to become independent of care again. Defining who will be the main caregiver is a dynamic and multifaceted process that can vary based on personal experiences and the sociocultural practices of each group or community in the settings where these families live (SANTOS, 2010).

The definition of who will be the caregiver initially comes from family arrangements, in an attempt to find "the right person" to take on this role. However, for cultural reasons, the role of caregiver for the elderly ends up falling mainly to daughters and spouses. This aspect could be observed in this investigation, as eight of the caregivers were women: wife, daughter, mother, and only two were men: husbands.

Despite the established changes, it was observed that caregivers carry with them values and customs related to the role of the family, linked to the responsibility of having to take care of a sick family member, being responsible for that person, especially when it is perceived that they are suffering some impairment in their physical integrity due to a lack of care. The caregiver's values and customs were manifested and originated from their daily life, from their relationships in the cultural context in which they are inserted and, from there, the **assumption of the role of main caregiver** can be seen, which can be confirmed in the following excerpt:

In fact, my mother was married twice, and with her second husband they lived in the countryside, on a farm, but my stepfather became ill, had a stroke, so they ended up coming here, first they lived with my sister, we are 7 children. What happened was this: I began to notice some "strange things" (Pause), when I went to visit my mother, she was happier, but when it was time to leave she wouldn't accept it, she insisted that I stay, so every time I left, I left crying, you know! So I told my sister who lives in Uberlândia that I was going to find a place to live with my mother, and she agreed, saying: that's right, it'll be good for her. (Dina)

It became clear during the interviews that the caregivers had a history of caring for other family members, or had worked as formal caregivers. The fact that they had **previous experience with the process of caring for another person/family member at home** seemed to favor their current care routine, giving them the security and autonomy to play the role of family caregiver.

I worked in a house where there were three people, one was blind, Mrs. "M", the other was an old lady, mute and deaf, and she had a brother, there were three brothers. "G" was deaf-mute, I would go there and arrange the house, everything for them, buy for them, he would ask me things I didn't understand, he would write them down for me, "A" would get there just by touching her and she would know it was me. It was God preparing me to take care of them, right?

Previous experience also stands out as a facilitating element in the process of adapting to the routine of care that needs to be offered to the current family member who is dependent on care, which can be seen in the following statements:

Sarah [daughter] was born with cerebral palsy and has never had any treatment, now that my son is doing physiotherapy on her, he's a physiotherapist [pause] I've always looked after them. (Adameire)

When my sister, when my brother, I looked after my sister, I lived in Benfica. I would leave Benfica, come here, clean the house, take her to the doctor, because I was the one who took her to the doctor, everywhere. We'd ask for a car over there, ask for a neighbor over here, because the neighbors here are, [stutters] crazy to do us favors. Then I'd pick her up, take her for hemodialysis, because she had a kidney problem, she couldn't have surgery because she was paralyzed and if you cut it, it won't heal. So I took her to the doctor, to hemodialysis, to take blood. That's how it was for about ten years with my sister. Then she passed away, it's been more than twenty years since she died. She passed away and I started looking after my father, my father was also always getting ill, I was always going out to take him to the doctor. I took him to the doctor, I took him to the bank, because I was also the one who got paid. Then, all of a sudden, because my father wasn't a troublemaker either, he got sick and we took him to the polyclinic, he stayed there for five hours, then he was transferred to Santa Casa for the night and the next day God took him away. (Lia)

But now he can't, but before that, during his mother's time, it was like that too, right Zaqueu [husband]? He had to take time off work, because I'm not very healthy, she suffered a stroke three times [her husband's mother], she had cerebral ischemia, and I, with my size [very short], would put her in the chair, come into the bathroom, give her a bath, change her diaper. I think she was in diapers for a year and seven months. Then, when she died, my mother was healthy and my father was too.

(Joshua)

From the moment that the elderly family caregiver takes on the integral care of their dependent elderly family member, they tend to give up their self-care needs in favor of the other, in other words, they start to **prioritize the needs of the being-caregiver.** Thus, the caregiver's self-care was no longer a priority among the elderly people surveyed and even their basic needs, such as bathing, were put on the back burner. The caregivers surveyed reported that they had no time to take care of their appearance or for leisure, which was observed in the following reports:

I live there taking care of them, I go to the doctor, I go for medicine at the clinic, I go to the doctor for them, I go for medicine, but there's nothing for me. (Lia)

So I have to prioritize her, first I do things for her and then I think about myself [pause], because today everything I do is for her. (Dina)

Pereira and Filgueiras (2009) emphasize that the caregiver, in addition to training to carry out certain types of care, needs planning that intervenes in their care and considers the overload they suffer, whether physical, psychological, financial or social, in order to promote the maintenance of their health.

In October it will be a year since he was admitted to [the public hospital] again. I stayed with him there day and night, it was very difficult, I slept in a chair. Then he went to [another public hospital], which was even worse. After that, I'm now paying for a hospitalization plan for him, but I don't need it, so he said I have to do it, but let it go, the important thing is you [referring to her husband] and you won't have to go through what you went through, it was too much noise.

Eunice's story drew our attention to the legal issue of health care for the elderly. According to chapter IV, article 15 of the Statute of the Elderly, comprehensive health care for the elderly is ensured through the SUS, guaranteeing universal and equal access, in an articulated and continuous set of actions and services, for the prevention, promotion, protection and recovery of health, including special attention to diseases that preferentially affect the elderly (BRASIL, 2003).

However, what we see is that, in order to guarantee adequate care, they believe they have to turn to the private health system, through health plans. In turn, health plans that provide comprehensive care, entitling them to outpatient consultations, exams and hospitalization, have abusive costs because, not infrequently, users suffer from chronic non-communicable diseases which, because they are considered pre-existing, end up being covered by shortages and justifying the non-coverage of expenses. Returning to legislation on health plans, art. 15, §3 of the Statute of the Elderly states that discrimination against the elderly in health plans by charging different amounts based on age is prohibited (BRASIL, 2012).

Faced with these issues, the elderly, even though they are protected by the country's current legislation, become fragile, as they are unable to receive comprehensive care from the SUS and, in order to take advantage of this care in the private sector, they will have to spend a significant portion of their income, even if they can afford to do so. In this study, five families use the private health system in some way, with priority being given to the family member being cared for; the other families use SUS care exclusively.

Another relevant issue that generated a code for the study was **changes in lifestyle related to the caring process,** which can be understood, in the perception of the study participants, as the aspects that influenced radical changes in their way of life from the moment they took on the care of their dependent family member. Elderly family caregivers described moving away from other family members, abandoning their religion and, above all, being unable to leave the house, as well as abandoning their home and leisure time.

In this way, with the restrictions imposed by day-to-day care, the caregiver stops doing activities that give them pleasure and well-being, such as physical activity, leisure and health care, prioritizing the care of the dependent family member to the detriment of self-care:

It's changed a lot, right! Because when it was just the two of us, we'd close the door and leave, right! We traveled a lot.

It was all very quick, I decided, I soon got a house in Marumbi, she didn't want to come here, my house is in Sao Judas, but then I left everything behind, my house, my children, everything really.... everything to take care of her, and since 2012 I've been taking care of her entirely. [pause] it's not easy, not because I like going out, it's not like that, in fact I've always been very homely, I prefer to stay at home, but the responsibility, right? [long pause]. As I said, I left everything behind, my children, and that's why I convinced us to move here, because here I'm closer to them, they were kind of thrown around, you know, not because I wanted to, but because I can't go out without her anymore, or leave her alone. (Dina)

Then the doctor advised that we would have to move out of that apartment, because it was difficult to go down and up the stairs, so it was very difficult for me to help go down and up, so we decided to move in, right, we moved into a house, there are no stairs, the car stops at the door, you just get in and out. [...] It's difficult for me, right, because I don't have a social life, it's difficult for me to go out. And today it's all changed, because if I go to the market, I have to leave him in bed and run back. If I go to the bank, I have to leave him in bed, I run." (Eunice)

So I said: I'm going to move there. Then I came here, talked to the older brothers, they said: you can move there, there's an empty house at the back, you won't have any expenses, you'll just have to look after your mother. (Lia)

A lot has changed, because then I lost what I had as a priority, which was my freedom to come and go. And today I no longer have that freedom, today I have to be limited to it. I can't say, "One hour from now I'm going to get on a bus and go to the city and do this and that", I can't do that. I know I can't. I have my responsibility, I had a hard time managing it, but little by little I came to terms with it, because it's day-to-day life that teaches you what your life is going to be like. (Gedeao)

It can be seen from the excerpts above that taking on the task of main caregiver means accepting a radical change in lifestyle. It involves everyday changes, such as the difficulty of going out to pay a bill, to the fact of having to give up your freedom, leisure and even the place where you live, due to the need for adjustments or for economic reasons. When the caregiver has a spouse, the change doesn't just occur in the life of the caregiver, but in the lives of both. They end up changing the routine they had in their married life, to the detriment of caring for their family member. And when they have children, the caregiver may experience a sudden change in the family arrangement, having to choose to stop living with their children on a daily basis in order to care for the dependent family member. On the other hand, some clearly demonstrate the contradictory feelings specified in the literature, see Ruth's excerpt:

It hasn't really changed much, because I've never been one to go out too much, God gives me strength, because I live in a jail without a wall (laughs without motivation). (Ruth)

For Elias (1985), the relationship between individuals and society is inseparable. Individuals are in a society formed by social relations and separated by an invisible barrier. It is necessary to understand human webs and, above all, the social configurations of each individual. The act of caring for others is complex and permeated by distinct and conflicting feelings (BRASIL, 2008b) and, on the other side, we have the person who depends on the care, also with the same contradictory feelings, which can make the relationship between caregiver and person being cared for conflicting. At the same time as the interviewee reports that she has not seen any major changes in her life, she says that God gives her strength, because she lives in a jail without walls, thus demonstrating a mixture of feelings that lead her to battles within herself, but that she places in a greater, supreme force that gives her the strength to carry on.

According to the Practical Guide for the Caregiver (BRASIL, 2008b), the change in daily activities, added to the care of the dependent family member, ends up overloading the caregiver, who may manifest physical tiredness, depression, abandonment of work, changes in marital and family life, depreciating not only himself, but also the person being cared for. Therefore, if these changes are not properly managed, they can cause the caregiver to become ill.

The process of caring for an elderly person at home can result in limitations in the daily life of the family caregiver, compromising their social, occupational and personal roles, with a consequent risk to their health and well-being. In the study in question, it was observed that the participating caregivers, without exception, are affected by at least one chronic non-communicable disease. The following are excerpts from statements which may confirm this

Compromised health of the elderly caregiver:

Just a few days ago, I got sick there, I ended up at the UPA, and the next thing you know I had a glucose level of 480, I have a glucose level, I have a diabetic problem, you know? (Lia)

I find it difficult, just like this week, I was feeling pain everywhere, but I don't know what I was feeling. (Adameire)

You know, I also have health problems, arthritis in my knees, but some days I don't walk well [brief pause], some days my legs hurt too much. (Ruth)

I have hypertension, I'm diabetic, I have a lot of pain in my body. I'm being treated by an endocrinologist because I have a thyroid problem, and it's very high. I'm taking medication that's higher than possible, the doctor said it's higher than my thyroid dosage, but now I've had a test and it's gone down a bit. It's been a year or so since the pain, the pressure and the thyroid started, it's about 6 years since I found out. (Eunice)

I have rheumatoid arthritis, I have two prostheses, I can't walk, I have problems with my blood pressure, but it's under control, thank God, everything is fine. (Isabel)

I have arthrosis in my feet, in my knees, I feel severe pain, it makes me almost unable to walk some days [...] I have a hemorrhoid problem, I have diverticulitis, reflux, hypertension [...] things of age, right?

Faced with compromised health and the odd responsibility of caring for another person, the caregiver starts to live with and even incorporate chronic illnesses into their way of life. They adapt to the health-disease process and organize themselves on a daily basis in order to meet the needs of the other person and, at the same time, to continue living within this new context.

5.7.2 Being a family caregiver and its implications for health and self-care

Aging is part of a natural and progressive process in the life cycle, which points to a stage of life made up of successive changes, including physical, mental and social, which arise from the natural wear and tear of bodily, psychological and cognitive structures. And when elderly people take on the role of family caregiver, the work can become more difficult.

This was perceived in the speeches, especially of the elderly women caregivers. They showed, during the observation and even during the interviews, that they get tired, but at the same time, they show positive feelings about the act of caring and that they will continue to care for as long as they live. And for this, they hope and believe in the power of a higher being who supports them and gives them strength.

It emerged that, because they carry with them values and customs related to the family role, when they take on the care of a sick family member, a reciprocal bond arises, transversal to the daily coexistence that leads to the difficulty of moving **away from the person being cared for, due to the bond of trust that is created between them,** both because of the difficulty of accepting the elderly person being cared for by someone else, and because of the caregiver's difficulty in trusting the ability of other family members to perform the function they carry out on a daily basis. This could be seen in some of the statements made by the main caregivers:

I go, but my head stays here, it's very difficult, it's changed a lot. Even though I leave my daughter here with him, I go, but I get worried, you know? I'm afraid he'll get sick and she won't know how to take care of him the way I do. (Eunice)

Like when I need to go out, I usually go out and I don't even say I'm going out, because if I say I'm going out he gets sick, he says I'm feeling ill, so we don't go out. And if I go out and he stays at home, he doesn't seem to miss it. If it doesn't take too long, he doesn't miss it. He doesn't stay alone.

And every time I get sick and tell her I'm going to the doctor, she panics, she won't let me. Oh no, don't go, I'm feeling ill and I can't stay here alone. Fear, she's afraid of being alone with him (referring to her brother with a mental disorder, who is also looked after by her).I encounter all sorts of difficulties, because if I leave the house I'm left with the two of them in my head, I have to keep them both inside to protect them. (Lia)

I say she's my family, I don't like to leave her alone, and she doesn't either. (Gedeao)

And he doesn't like accepting someone else either, it's difficult, complicated and now it's getting worse because his head is getting really bad, you've seen three strokes, right?

When analyzing the statements made by caregivers, it is important to highlight the importance of certain agreements between the caregiver and the person being cared for, in order to guarantee a certain degree of independence for both the caregiver and the person being cared for. An essential point for this agreement is the encouragement of self-care for both (BRASIL, 2008b). On the other hand, it is necessary to emphasize the issues related to social support or social networks, which would be composed of a structure and a function, which are distinct aspects and phenomena and which, as such, should be evaluated and examined (BOCCHI; ANGELO, 2008).

The structure of social relationships refers to the organization of the bond between individuals and can be described in various ways. The structure of social relationships is made up of a network of formal and informal relationships. Formal relationships are relationships maintained due to position and roles in society and include: health professionals, teachers, lawyers, among others. Informal social relationships - those considered to be of greater personal and affective importance than the more specialized and formal relationships - are made up of all individuals (family, friends, neighbors, work colleagues, community) and the link between individuals with whom one has a close family relationship or affective involvement (DUE *et al.*, 1999).

From the moment that caregivers feel insecure about leaving the house, leaving their loved one for a few moments, there is an idea of a lack of social support received on a daily basis. The social support provided effectively serves as an intervening factor in the quality of life of the family caregiver-family caregiver binomial, by giving the family member some freedom to resume part of their previous life in the role of caring fully for another person.

Weaknesses in carrying out the role of caregiver were defined as the family caregiver not being able to carry out the activity that the person being cared for requires, the fact that they are also elderly, suffering from a pathology or simply not being able to carry out the tasks due to their own aging process.

I have to push myself, then I feel a lot of pain... (Ruth)

I was afraid of her falling, falling, then I was afraid of her getting worse, but she's too heavy for me. (Adameire)

Ah, I don't know, there are times when I wonder, you know? There are times when I wonder: it's too much pressure for me, it's too tiring, having to look after her, him, my youngest daughter. (Lia)

Some days we worry, people! Will I be able to cope? But I think to myself, Our Lady passes by, she'll help me, and off she goes rowing, right?

When he was in bed and needed to go to the bathroom, which I couldn't take him to, I have a son who would come over from time to time to help out, but not always, because he has his own house, sometimes I would ask the guy from the garage or the neighbor to come over and put him in the bath chair, to give him a bath, and I couldn't either, because I have a serious health problem [at this point he showed me his feet with deformities due to arthrosis]. (Talita)

The speeches allow us to evaluate what the elderly do about their care process: they find the task difficult and tiring. We therefore realize that they need help with this responsibility. Therefore, the inference is that family and professional support with encouragement, whether through nursing consultations, educational groups or home visits, with a view to self-care, can be provided to this population, in order to promote the exchange of experiences between participants, encouraging positive practices and adjusting negative ones through clear and simple language.

The **lack of time** emphasized proved to be an important detrimental factor to the self-care of caregivers, who end up neglecting their health, physical appearance, clothing, leisure and personal well-being. In this way, the quality of life of family caregivers suffers if their basic needs are not met, as well as their needs for pleasure, well-being and personal and spiritual fulfillment, which, as can be seen in the reports, end up being sacrificed as a result of becoming caregivers. With the change in routine and, consequently, in the caregiver's life, they come up against other difficulties that distance them from self-care, such as the increase in time spent caring for their dependent family member. The caregivers reported that they have to spend a lot of time on their job, thus reducing their time for self-care:

The workload has increased, looking after elderly people isn't easy. I used to look after my health and now I don't have the time. (Lia)

When I call my daughter to go to school, she gets up at 5:30 in the morning, can you imagine! Yesterday I went to bed at 1 a.m. (Lia)

He says I have to do water aerobics and walk. Doctor, what am I going to do? Walk for 40 minutes, 20 minutes. I can't stand it, with my whole body, all this weight. To go for a walk, go downhill, and when it's time to go up, I'm going to have a heart attack, he doesn't understand, there's no time left. (Eunice)

This subcategory brought to light the critical situations or obstacles that family caregivers face. It was noted that care for the body, sleep, food and health are deficient, due to lack of time and the absence of another person who can "take over" from the family caregiver. This once again brings up the issue of the caregiver being able to count on social support.

No, I don't have a pressure problem, I used to have a pressure problem only when I got nervous, it's like this nervous state, that anxiety, that nervousness, then it would go up. I don't take anything for blood pressure anymore, only for diabetes. I don't know if it's improved either, it was too high, I've got to find some time, I've got to work on it. (Lia)

The **deficit of leisure time** is a constant in the lives of the caregivers who took part in the study, based on the fact that there is little or no leisure time activity in the daily routine of the caregiver, who reports not being able to do the activities they have always enjoyed. In fulfilling their roles, family caregivers stop doing various activities they enjoy, such as traveling, going to church, watching TV, going out or talking to friends, which characterizes a leisure deficit on the part of these caregivers and can be analyzed from the excerpts of the interviews that follow:

What's changed is that I don't care much about going out, I don't make friends, I don't have a social life, I have a life just for them. I don't even go to my daughter's house, she lives here in Juiz de Fora. (Adameire)

Yesterday, he [referring to his husband] went on a trip, he's already been on two trips without me, because, at first, we didn't go out alone, we only went out together, we went to the beach. When I had my mother, we went to the beach. One day we went to Piùma, we stayed there for a fortnight, so we didn't have that responsibility, right? Not now, I go, he stays, he goes, I stay [laughs, without motivation]. (Joshua)

The following excerpts from the interviews with Adameire and Eunice allowed us to understand how they had to stop attending their religious beliefs to the detriment of caring for two dependent elderly people, their daughter and her husband, in the case of one, and her husband, in the case of the other:

You know, I didn't leave because I wanted to, there's nothing like that, because I didn't leave out of spite, I didn't leave because I stopped being, I left because I couldn't afford to go (pause). I used to work [referring to the Spiritist Center meetings I attended] in the city center, every Monday, Friday and Saturday. (Adameire)

No, I don't do anything anymore, because before I used to go to church, but I'm not even going to church, it's not possible with him like this. (Eunice)

The above comments bring us back to the issue of the elderly having their spirituality/religiosity developed. Many elderly people stop attending services, masses, etc., linked to their religious affiliation, due to various factors, including the difficulty of access and worsening health conditions. In the case of this study, to the detriment of the act of caring and not having someone to leave their loved one with so that they can continue doing this activity, which for them also functions as a leisure activity.

The **activities carried out by the elderly family caregiver** that emerged during the investigation point to the need for support for the elderly family caregiver, by nurses and other health professionals, in order to provide better conditions for caring for the dependent elderly, as well as security for the caregiver, who needs knowledge and skills to carry out the role delegated to them. This family member needs to be prepared and accompanied in the performance of this new role of caregiver, helping them to overcome difficulties and provide quality care that meets the needs identified and is equivalent to the family's cultural context. This will contribute to the process of adaptation in the performance of care activities, as well as self-care.

During the interviews, it emerged that caregivers carry out care activities without any training or monitoring by health professionals, as can be seen in the following excerpts:

I'm the one who applies the insulin, does the blood sugar and checks my BP every day. (Gedeao)

At night, he often gets sick, his pressure rises, it goes to 18, then his heart rate goes to 110, 130, I give him another pill for his pressure, I put cold towels on his forehead, he gets very hot. Then he cools down and gets over it." (Eunice)

According to the Ministry of Health's Practical Guide for Caregivers, the caregiver's role is to accompany and assist the person being cared for, doing for them only what they are unable to do on their own. Techniques and procedures that are characteristic of legally established professions, particularly in the nursing field, are not part of their routine (BRASIL, 2008b).

The other activities carried out by elderly caregivers that were identified during the home visit and in excerpts from family members' statements in the interviews consist of administering medication, giving or helping with bathing, brushing teeth, helping to go to the bathroom, promoting leisure and spiritual activities, searching for health materials and care, and caring for the integrity of the skin and preventing injuries, etc.

I give her lunch, I put her in the bath, because I like to help her put her clothes on, because it's so she doesn't get too tired, because she has fibrosis in her lungs too, so she doesn't get too tired, so I help her put her clothes on, but she bathes herself, I just help her put her clothes on, I put cream on her legs, because she has a varicose vein problem, a serious one too, so she has to be well moisturized, because otherwise it's a problem. (Isabel)

I have to do everything: bathe her, feed her, give her medicine. She eats on her own, but she spills it, half of it on her lap, but she eats, and she goes to the bathroom and pees on her own, sometimes to clean up after herself, when she poops, then she calls me. (Lia)

Over the last year he's gotten a lot worse, he's even started drooling... and he doesn't want to sit still, so if he goes one way, I go too, if he goes the other way, I follow. (Ruth)

Of the ten participants, eight reported that the accumulation of daily tasks leads to physical and mental fatigue, which can be detrimental to the care process, as there are many domestic tasks to be carried out on a daily basis, such as washing and ironing clothes, cooking, tidying the house, among others, and not simply caring for the family member. This has led to the code **maintenance of the house and the environment in which they live with the elderly person,** which, for them, is all the daily activities involved in caring for the environment at the same time, creating an overload.

And I'm the one who does all the chores: I do the laundry, tidy up the house, make the food, as well as looking after him. (Ruth)

I do the washing, I don't do the ironing, whoever wants their clothes ironed, they do it, right? I used to do it when I was young. I make lunch, I only make lunch, I heat it up for dinner, if you want I make soup. (Adameire)

Food has to be freshly prepared, she can't cook, so I do everything. Likewise, after I moved in, I still haven't managed to do that cleaning [everything is clean, looks great, very organized]. (Dina)

Like cleaning the house, I started cleaning the house last Monday, I did the bathroom, then on Tuesday I did the kitchen, you know! When it was Wednesday I did her room, Friday I did the living room, it's like this, every day I do something, because I can't do everything at once and she won't let me either, you know! (Lia)

So I'm the one who's there 24 hours a day, there's no way, I'm the one who has to go to the street with all my difficulties, I have to go to the street to pay bills, I do everything, I cook, I just don't clean the house, because she does it every Monday [referring to her unmarried daughter, who lives with them but works all day], so it's up to her, the rest I do. (Talita)

It's clear from the speeches that the routine activities, or rather, the accumulation of tasks on their part, makes it difficult for them to exercise self-care, leading to compromised health. This increase in daily activities, the sudden changes in routine and the family caregiver's responsibility for caring for the dependent family member, as well as household chores, make it difficult for them to fully perform self-care. Another point to note among the participants was that they are very demanding of themselves in terms of cleanliness and, even though the house was in adequate hygiene conditions, some reported that it was not as clean as it should be.

5.8 FAMILY SUPPORT

This category brings to light the concept that, in addition to the family caregiver having undergone the changes in their life context analyzed above, which directly interfere in the process of caring for others. It is understood that, as the family caregiver takes charge of their relative's care at home, the care process and self-care will be influenced by the stimuli from the rest of the family. The family caregiver's ties with other family members vary between favorable (positive) and unfavorable (negative) aspects, which were addressed in this category through the following subcategories: "family support, positively influencing the process of caring for the other" and "the absence of family support, negatively influencing the caregiver's health".

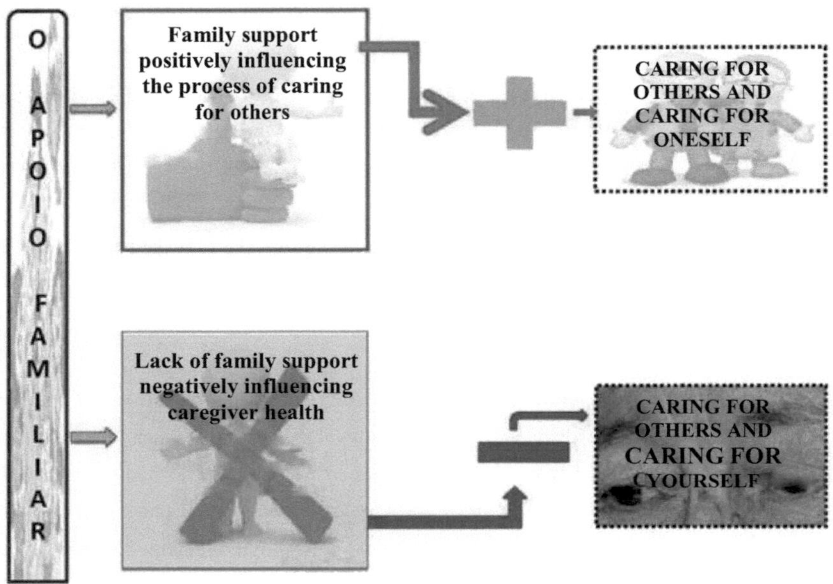

5.8.1 Family support positively influencing the process of caring for others

The elderly family caregiver's life context is marked by interactions with close people: family and friends, whose influence becomes clear from the data. Sometimes in a positive way, as a support and encouraging element; at other times, in opposition, the lack of support, negatively influencing the whole process of caring for others and, consequently, self-care and, finally, affecting the health of the caregiver.

The workload on the caregiver is sometimes significant and, as was seen in the analysis of the previous category, the process of caring for the elderly in the home becomes routine as a result of the rapid ageing process and this process of caring without family support can lead to negative repercussions for physical and mental health, which will be reflected in the quality of life and well-being of both the caregivers and those being cared for. The participants in this study generally pointed out the importance of the presence of family, in the subcategory of **support received from family to care for others and self-care**, and expressively spoke about the help of family for support and improvement of quality of life conditions in general. The importance of family support was present in the interviewees' statements:

The basis of our lives is our family, right, below God is our family. So it's one sharing with the other so as not to weigh them down. [...] Sometimes, if I say today I need to go to the doctor, but then I have to see: doesn't he have to leave? Because if he has to leave, I can't. So we're always sharing, sometimes, even today I asked him: do you have to go out tomorrow? He said: I think I have to go out, but tomorrow is also my church day, so I'll go later. (Joshua)

My whole family loves him, my daughter worries too much, she's having a problem at home with her husband, with illness too. But she cares a lot, she comes here whenever she can. There are the grandchildren, a beautiful great-granddaughter, with blue eyes, thank God everything's going well, nobody's turned to anything, to drugs, everything's at university, they don't like *funk,* anything, so this gives us a lot of peace of mind. (Eunice)

As time went by, they realized that she had lost weight, because the doctor had already said that she couldn't put on weight, I took care of her diet, she didn't sleep like she used to, she was sleeping all day with my sister. [I don't want to speak ill of her, but [pause]. She'd get up just to eat, take her medicine, she was already giving off that bad smell, even of urine, which sometimes escapes, and if you don't wash it off, right! Then, after they started to realize that she was getting better, they started to come back, but my brother didn't [showed sadness and resentment]. (Dina)

The reports show that caregivers who receive continuous and assisted family support are able to reduce their time caring for the other, contributing to a reduction in physical overload, leading to a reduction in anxiety when performing their role, favoring the **preserved self-care of the elderly caregiver**:

I go to the doctor: the same, Monday, I have a doctor at noon. My daughter comes and stays with her. (Isabel)

Like, for example, last week I needed to go to the doctor, I had to be there at 7 o'clock at Joao Penido, so my daughter stayed with her. [...] I don't know much about it here yet, but I've been to the clinic, talked to the nurse, [...], I even told her that I wanted referrals to ACISPES, since I can already be seen there, right? And I'm dying to have a CT scan, a densitometry." (Dina)

And the day I have to go to the doctor, he stays [referring to his husband], so I know I can go out carefree, too!" (Joshua)

In Gedeao's account, as observed in the testimonies of other elderly people, it can be seen that self-care, the will to look after oneself and the will to live have to come from oneself and, according to him, from a sacred force. They need to be well, because the other is already dependent. So one needs to be well in order to look after both. Isabel adds that doing activities that give pleasure removes negative feelings about the process of health and illness. And there are also reports, as in Joshua's case, of those who use integrative and complementary practices as allies in the process of ageing well.

In the scientific literature, one comes across different names for therapeutic practices. Alternative and complementary medicine has been defined as a group of different medical and health care systems, as well as practices that are not present in biomedicine (NATIONAL CENTER OF COMPLEMENTARY AND ALTERNATIVE MEDICINE, 2007), for which, in Brazil, the term integrative and complementary practices (PIC) is used. These include traditional Chinese medicine (especially acupuncture), homeopathy and anthroposophy, medicinal plants (phytotherapy) and social thermalism (crenotherapy) (BRASIL, 2006c).

Today I go out for 5 hours, I do water aerobics, I do it 3 times a week, I've been doing it for over a year.

If I have to go to the doctor, I don't make any effort. If I have to go, I go, and she goes with me. If I go to the urologist or the cardiologist, she goes with me. As far as possible, I take care of myself, I have a preventive prostate exam every year, last year I had a prostate ultrasound, I went to the urologist, this year I haven't been yet, because they haven't asked, but I'm already worried and I'm going to ask them to refer me again the day I go. I think this is important, I always talk to her, we can't both fall, someone has to be standing up to take care of the other. Because she's already dependent, if I become dependent too, what will our lives be like? There's no way. (Gedeao)

If someone stays with him, I can go out, go to the doctor. He goes too, [referring to her husband]. We take care of our health too, but we have to plan. This week I have to go to the doctor, we treat at homeopathy too, then when it's scheduled it has to be changed, one on one day and the other on the next. I have a lot of faith in homeopathy, because it doesn't hurt. I take valerian, mine is three in one, it's valerian, chamomile and there's another name for it, a stronger one. (Joshua)

I'm always at the doctor's looking to get better, but sometimes I don't go because I'm lazy, it's the age thing. But thank God, God has been giving me the strength to get as far as I have, because if he hadn't given me this strength, I would have given up by now. (Talita)

From this perspective, Eliopoulos (2011), in his study, showed that the majority of elderly people have internal resources, including physical, emotional and spiritual resources, which allow them to develop well in this phase of life, with the practice of activities that support self-care. The behaviors that exemplify their potential are, for example, assuming responsibility for self-care; mobilizing internal and external resources to develop strategies, solve problems and deal with moments of crisis, especially those related to health; recognizing and accepting the reality that life includes positive and negative events; and recognizing limitations and potential.

It has been observed that the elderly caregiver needs help from someone at various times to help them with certain tasks, or even so that they can go out to do something, such as going to the market or to the bank, or even for appointments, exams, etc. The **need** then arises **for support from a secondary caregiver, taking** turns which, even if only for a short time, helps to reduce the caregiver's burden:

So, when I feel a lot of pain and I'm not well, I end up having to ask for help, I'm afraid of letting him fall. (Isabel)

Like, today, you saw, I got a girl to give me a bath [she was leaving her house, when we arrived for the visit], I have to go there to explain the bath business and sometimes I don't even give the bath properly, it's just the bath that sacrifices me. [pause] It's going to be really hard for me to go to this doctor, because I have to leave someone with the people here, right? (Adameire)

So when I have to go, my daughter stays with him. Luckily, she doesn't work. She has a health problem, so she's on INSS benefits. So she puts her daughter in school and stays here with him. (Eunice)

If I need to go out, depending on what I'm doing, I need someone to stay with her. (Dina)

5.8.2 Lack of family support negatively influencing the health of the caregiver

From the observations made in the homes of the elderly, it could be seen that caregivers need to provide specific care at home in order to maintain and promote the health of the family member being cared for, as well as their own. The absence of family support has a negative influence on the health of the caregiver, which was evident in the case of the study participants, who are also elderly. We can see from their speech and expressions that, for them, family presence is of fundamental importance. I was able to understand that, at this stage of life, they are more reflective, emotional, like to talk and be listened to; they feel very devalued and saddened by the absence of their loved ones.

It was clear from the data and observations that the elderly family caregiver who looks after a dependent elderly person dedicates themselves entirely to the task, usually without the help of other family members. This direct exposure, over time, contributes to a greater risk of illness, deficits in self-care, physical overload and emotional discomfort. It was observed that the lack of help from other family members most of the time is a recurring report and emphasized, above all, by the **low or no family support.** The difficulty in getting support in dividing up the tasks of caring for the elderly may be associated with the fact that other family members work, but the reason seems to be the gap in the involvement of other family members with the elderly person's situation of dependency and health problems. During the interviews, the interviewees were emotional:

The test results will come back, but I'll have to book a doctor.

It's going to be really hard for me to go to this doctor [pause, showing sadness]. I don't have my brothers anymore, I used to have nine. My mother! I'm married for the second time, Sarah is the eldest, the daughter from my first marriage. He's alone too, just the two of us and the kids now, right, but they work...right!" (Adameire)

It's just the two of us here! Just the two of us [referring to her husband], just the three of us [referring to her husband and the father she cares for]. No one else helps.

His children don't have any contact with him, they live in Rio, but since he split up, his mother has made intrigues and they don't like him. When I married him, I tried everything to bring them back together, I called them to come over for lunch, but there was no way. I think he's really sorry about that, especially now, around Christmas, right?

[...] I'm retired, she's retired too, so God blesses her and gives her enough to live on, but personal help like this is very difficult, because when we lived together with her daughter, it was enough, barely, but it helped, but today I can't even stay here with her to go to the doctor. To go, I have to take her with me [pause]. If I'm going to do anything, I have to take her, because there's no one to stay here. (Gedeao)

I'm 79 and he's 81. So it's complicated for me, because I'm at the stage where I need a caregiver, but I can't afford one, because a caregiver doesn't come cheap. I know it's more than one salary. And they [referring to their children] work, right?

One of the participants reported that family members "disappear" for fear of being held responsible for the care in some way. Watch:

Look, it's a big responsibility, right, because I'm alone [pause]. I don't get anything, there are some who don't even call, because they know there's going to be a problem. Oh, she'll complain, she'll ask for this, she'll ask for that. There's one who came here when my father died. My father is fifteen years old, there's one who lives here in Juiz de Fora, the one who hasn't called for fifteen years is the one who lives in Belo Horizonte. She's married and her husband is a councillor. We had 11 siblings, then four died and seven were left, of those seven, me [she stuttered again, showing high anxiety] and my brother, Lucas and the other five don't care, there are three male siblings and two female siblings. And there's a female sister who lives here in Juiz de Fora, in Furtado de Menezes, you know? But she doesn't care either, she doesn't look, she doesn't want to know, you know? So it's very difficult to deal with the situation, sometimes I'm even disgusted, when I see her, when I take her to have a bath, I see her little body all transformed, you know? [pause, I cry] it revolts me, it revolts me to see [a tearful cry begins, with enormous suffering, which moved me deeply, I felt like crying along], the children don't care about her, it's just on my back. I suffer from seeing her suffer [a lot of sadness and revolt at the lack of family support]. (Lia)

Lia's speech once again reminds us of the need for support for the caregiver through social networks. Often, caregivers do not have adequate support to assist the family member they are caring for. Social support from the family itself is essential for maintaining the care of elderly people suffering from incapacitating illnesses. In the absence of support and relevant guidance, the family caregiver is led to physical and mental overload, an intervening factor that contributes to the impairment of the quality of life of the elderly caregiver-elderly family member binomial.

Gedeao's speech helps us understand how the family plays an essential role in maintaining life and reducing the physical and emotional strain on this couple:

I think that if the family were united like this, if they held hands, shared, it would be easier, but as this is almost impossible, I think it's difficult to achieve anything to improve this living condition. Because when you have one plus one, that's two. The load becomes lighter, but this other side is difficult to achieve, so [paused]. Family is everything, under God it's everything, because if you have the support of family, you can trust the person to leave you, if you have their daughter, I'll leave more relaxed because I know I can trust them, I don't need to be stressed wherever I go, if it takes two or three hours, if I leave someone who isn't family, first of all I won't be free to leave my house in the hands of someone who [pause]. If it's not family it's difficult, but family is united when it comes to having parties, barbecues, winning things, then it's united, but in the rest it's not united.

In addition to the lack of family support, a **family conflict** code emerged from the data, related to the role of the main caregiver. Families don't want to take on the family member's full care, but when a family member is willing to play the role of family caregiver, this generates conflicts, mainly due to financial aspects, i.e. they don't want to take on the care, but they want to enjoy the income that the elderly person has acquired in their lifetime.

But (pause) [voice breaking], with this, me looking after her directly, my family got upset with me, they thought, and one of my brothers even said, that I was only doing this out of interest in my mother's pension, or rather, her pensions, right! You see, she has two pensions, one from her husband's FUNRURAL and another because she worked a lot and retired. [...] You know, this brother of mine, he's the one I got on with the most, we were very close and I decided to take care of my mother, he was the one who accused me the most, after that, he never came here again, he told me that if I meet him in the street, if I'm on one side of the street I'd better cross, and if I pass in the street and he's with his truck he'll drive over me, wow, it hurts, it hurts too much, this is very difficult for me [silence]. Now I don't understand why he acts like that, but one day, God willing, it will pass. (Dina)

The research data shows that the elderly person continues to provide for the family in part or in full with their retirement, even when they depend on the full care of a caregiver who, in the case of this study, is also elderly and may or may not have some kind of income of their own. When the caregiver takes on full care and becomes responsible for the elderly person's care, this can trigger a family crisis because of the caregiver's income. Some family members don't want to take on the care, but want to take advantage of the elderly person's personal income in some way, as a way of guaranteeing all or part of their subsistence. As a consequence, the initial logic of the act of caring will be reversed, with the elderly person no longer being the object of care, but the one who guarantees care, both for them and their family members.

In other cases, the elderly person's income may not be enough to support themselves, a situation from which the **economic aspects** code was deduced, which is related to the increase in costs and the family budget, indicating cases in which the caregiver reported an increase in the cost of providing care, either with medication or with any type of treatment for the dependent family member.

His money isn't even enough to buy the medicine, it's a lot of medicine... (Adameire)

And there's a physiotherapist who comes every week, every Friday at 6:30 in the afternoon, because I can't do it more often, it would have to be more than once, to take him to hydrotherapy, but I can't. I'd have to have a car, a man to go with me to take him. (Talita)

While some elderly people continue to provide for their families, there were situations in which, due to health problems and chronic conditions that cost a lot, they are unable to support themselves, depending on the help of other family members. The financial difficulties resulting from low purchasing power, concomitant with the increase in expenses due to the demands of the process of caring for others and their own health, such as the need to buy medicines that are not provided by the SUS and the specific demands of care, could be observed in the daily lives of some elderly people.

The concern about financial support for self-care, added to other aspects, contributes to physical and emotional exhaustion, as it is another element that generates concern in the context of care at home. The reports show that, even though they had a monthly income, in the event of financial need due to illness, the elderly people surveyed reported that they had nowhere else to turn, increasing their concern about the well-being of the dependent elderly person. In this way, a proposition can be made about the health work process. It is important that health professionals take care to adapt the care plan to the individuality and context of each elderly person, so that it is a real plan that can be carried out by these individuals.

There is also a factor that is close to the previous one and contributes greatly to the physical and emotional strain on the elderly caregiver, which is when they become **financially dependent on another family member**.

I can't afford it, I haven't retired. It's like this, it's going to be very bad, but I have to say it. T", my daughter, who is a tax inspector for [...], a tax auditor for the federal revenue service, she put Sarah and me down as her dependents, because she was a very sick girl [referring to her daughter Sarah], she even had tuberculosis in her bones, it took a lot to heal, at that time tuberculosis was a seven-headed beast, right? And she had it, and because of that, we can't retire and get our money, so she buys it, and pays for the health plan [pause] of the one that only treats hospitalization, and it's very expensive, right, and the older we get, she doesn't let us lack much comfort [lack of motivation in this speech].

(Adameire)

And in this case, the caregiver, who even though elderly, has no income of their own, becomes dependent on other family members, which many consider to be ideal, but which, for the elderly person, is not what they expect. In another case, during the family arrangements to find a family member to be the caregiver, benefits are guaranteed by the other family members. Take a look:

Then I said: but are you going to help me look after my mother? Because going there to look after her alone, I'm going to need some money, because I won't be able to work, so they said, we'll see about that later, I mean, I've been here for four years now. [...] because the family, the brothers don't help me financially with anything. (Lia)

In the case of Lia, who gave up her way of life and her job to look after her family member, she found herself without help from her family, both in terms of care and financial support. See the excerpt below:

I haven't been able to retire yet, because I don't have the time, you know! I worked, but a lot of people didn't contribute to my INPS, a lot of the houses I worked in, family homes, and things, so they didn't pay the INPS, so I was left without the INPS, now I'm looking for it, to see if I can at least pull over, so I can have my earnings, right, my money, because I'm going to use my mother's and my brother's money, that's not good. I have to have my own so I can look after my daughter. Because she needs a lot of things, and I can't give them to her. (Lia)

Couto's (2013) study on family caregivers of dependent elderly people included in subcategories the abandonment of work in order to care, within the experiences of being a caregiver for a dependent elderly person, and showed that this was a negative aspect, in the subjects' conception, as they end up considering that they no longer have a "life of their own", leading even to social isolation.

In the view of the study participants, they consider that, as they are routinely deprived of family support, they may suffer from insecurity related to urban violence, which configures the topic of **feeling unprotected and afraid of violence.**

And there's something else I'm afraid of (crying), this low wall, things the way they are, nobody respects anyone, these things [...]I'm afraid of someone coming in with bad intentions, us here alone, for example, here was his workshop, when he stopped working he couldn't walk inside it, so much iron on the ground, now he goes there to see if he can find a piece of iron. They took everything, even all the tools." (Adameire)

When I go out, I have to lock them both in the house, I close the outside door and take the key, because if I leave the door open, everyone who calls out will put them in the house, they have no sense, neither he nor she, understand? And we can't play, can we?" (Lia)

The situation pointed out by the caregivers is related to what was found in a study carried out by the Federal University of Juiz de Fora in 2012, in which the elderly interviewed listed their most frequent fear as being related to safety, fear of violence (UNIVERSIDADE FEDERAL DE JUIZ DE FORA, 2012).

At the same time as they feel they have little family support, the elderly generally want to maintain their independence, because they don't want to show that they end up needing help to carry out activities, even everyday household chores. This gives rise to a **sense of apprehension at being considered a burden on the family**, as the elderly think that they should solve problems and carry out activities with as much autonomy as possible, because their relatives work and have families. Thus, the elderly believe that they should only turn to them when they have no other way of resolving everyday situations or even those that are unexpected:

I try not to call his children, it's because I have six stepchildren, "L" was seven when we got married, she's the one who lives in front. [...] They help, but you know, they all have families, children, husbands and they live far away, so "L" is the one who helps the most, she also has her grandchildren, but I try to do what I can, only when I can't stand it, because Lane helps a lot, but she has her children, her husband, she has her own life, right?

In 2012, 2011, he became ill, he had crises every day, his blood pressure rose, and I was alone with him. Then my daughter said: call me and I'll come. Then I said: but what are you going to do? He doesn't want me to call, he won't [the husband says]. Let's go to the doctor, I don't want to, you're going to look after me, it'll go down and right now I'm fine. (Eunice)

What's missing is that it's not possible to solve everything, because she [referring to one of her daughters] didn't get married, but decided to raise other people's children, and her daughters are three, all three have problems, one had a child when she was 15 and now she has three children and the other two, who are twins, have problems like that, they don't reason, one doesn't reason at all, nothing, nothing and the other still reasons a little. [...] Then, with these children, she has to give little, and then the grandchildren come along, so she has to cut back, she's now cutting back on that whim she used to have with us. She doesn't let us lack anything, but she doesn't have that whim either, you can see the house as it is, we don't live in a house like this because we want to! Her house is very beautiful, but I don't go there either. (Adameire)

From these comments, it emerges that, at a certain point, the elderly person may no longer be able to look after themselves as they used to; they need help. In this sense, the ideal is for the family to meet with the elderly caregiver and the elderly person being cared for to define the best way forward and thus find accessible solutions, without the elderly having to sacrifice themselves quietly, avoiding asking for the presence of others, so as not to appear incapable of continuing to be independent. What I could see from the family caregiver's words, gestures and non-verbal communication is that they feel like a burden to the family, thus increasing their suffering unnecessarily. In other words, they perform the noble task of caring for another person on a daily basis, but they feel undervalued and in the background by the rest of the family.

In his study on the self-care of family caregivers of dependent adults or elderly people after hospital discharge, Costa (2012) observed that the deficit in the caregiver's self-care was related to difficulties in reconciling self-care with the care activities of the dependent family member. The finding **of difficulty in self-care** is directly related to the lack of family support.

And in the four years that I've been here, I've never been to the doctor again, preventive exams, mammograms, I've never been anymore, I don't take care of my health anymore.

So I haven't washed my head, so I keep scratching my head, worrying that I haven't washed my head, but I say, I'm not going to worry, otherwise I'll get sick. (Adameire)

My child! I've been going to the pharmacy for about three years now, after that I just buy my blood pressure medication, sometimes my blood pressure gets too high, then I go to the pharmacy, the girl looks at my blood pressure and that's it. (Ruth)

It is important that the elderly are encouraged and supported by their families and health professionals in terms of motivation for healthy ageing and, above all, for self-care and care at home.

In the participants' view, sadness is a human feeling that expresses discouragement and frustration at what is happening to oneself or to the person being cared for. It can be manifested through crying, insomnia, depression, lack of appetite, among others. And it can be perceived in the reports by the participants' expression **of sadness.**

There's no way, [crying] because now, both he and I and Sarah have to wait for death, there's no way [pause with crying, disconsolate], our time has passed, I'm not sad about it, I'm overwhelmed, because I'm just [pause] waiting for the end [silence, showing a lot of sadness]. (Adameire)

Sometimes I go to the yard to cry, sometimes I go to the back, right? Because I don't want to cry near my daughter, right? Sometimes she sees me and asks: what's wrong with you, mom, are you sick? She's only thirteen, right? And she has no idea, she suffers with me [eyes filled with tears]. One day she said: let's get out of here, mom, get me out of here, because he got nervous there overnight [referring to her brother, whom she also looks after], there's no way, right? Life is very difficult, very complicated." (Lia)

The situations experienced by caregivers can lead them to develop tension in relation to the role of caregiver, which is included among the nursing diagnoses proposed by the NANDA (North American Nursing Diagnoses Association) taxonomy, found in domain seven, referring to roles in relationships; in class one: caregiver roles. Hence the definition "difficulty performing the role of caregiver" (NORTH AMERICAN NURSING DIAGNOSIS ASSOCIATION, 2010).

Fernandes and Garcia (2009) identified the attributes of stress in family caregivers of dependent elderly people, when they surveyed the bio-psycho-social alterations suffered by family members, coming to the conclusion that family caregivers had alterations in their physical and emotional state, as well as an imbalance between activity and rest and compromised individual coping.

The authors revealed that the family caregiver was exposed to multiple types of stressors over a long period of time and ended up running the risk of presenting health problems similar to those of the person being cared for. The family caregiver is restricted in their own life by taking on the care to ensure the physical and psychosocial well-being of the person being cared for, and the burden related to this care means that the caregiver can also be seen as a client in need of care (FERNANDES; GARCIA, 2009).

From the interviewees' excerpts, it is possible to perceive the **physical overload of the elderly caregiver's role:**

I keep waiting for night to come so I can go to bed... (Ruth)

I sleep like a bird, I wake up several times to check on her. (Dina)

It is also possible to perceive the **emotional overload of the elderly caregiver's role**:

I'm already sick too, whatever I consider myself to be, because I consider myself to be sick, because I feel a lot of pain, pain all over my body, it's very difficult [shows deep sadness, remains silent, cries, voice bottled up], but we'll see, it's fine [another pause, thoughtful] I think it's very difficult [voice bottled up, again sadness and tears]. I feel a lot of sadness [cried a lot]. (Adameire)

So it's a struggle [...] Everything like that, right? Her body is damaged, because she also worked, she also struggled to raise us, in the fields, right, because we lived in the fields, she struggled, she cut sugar cane, together with me, with my father [she started to show a lot of emotion in her voice and her eyes shone], she planted corn, beans, all this she did in the fields to help raise us. Then I look at her little body, sitting there in that chair to take a bath with that body all deformed, you know, it revolts me [desperate crying]. (Lia)

From the data, it can be understood that the overload is outlined as routine due to the overlapping of tasks, the accumulation of activities, low family support and shortcomings in the health system, which make it impossible for this caregiver and the family member being cared for to have dignified and comprehensive health care. Economic and housing issues can also trigger the process of strain on the caregiver's role. In addition, the lack of preparation and the level of knowledge that the caregiver has about the care activities they carry out contribute to tension, stress and damage to the caregiver's quality of life.

Nurses therefore need to reflect on the various family structures, roles and relationships, in addition to identifying the self-care capacity of elderly caregivers, so that they can work more efficiently when faced with the need for specific nursing care for these elderly people at home (SANTOS, 2014).

5.9 ELDERLY CAREGIVER WHO TAKES CARE OF A DEPENDENT ELDERLY PERSON ON A DAILY BASIS, HEALTH AND THE HEALTH TEAM.

The fourth category brought up a contemporary and relevant discussion, based on Brazilian legislation, which today is seen as a public health issue, since, as a result of the ageing process, as explained above, chronic non-communicable diseases arise and, in the case of this study, we have the elderly caregiver/dependent elderly binomial. The caregiver who takes on the full burden of care therefore needs institutionalized support from a multi-professional team. The emphasis in this study will be on nurses.

DIAGRAM 5 - THE ELDERLY CAREGIVER WHO TAKES CARE OF AN ELDERLY PERSON AT HOME ON A DAILY BASIS AND THE HEALTH TEAM.

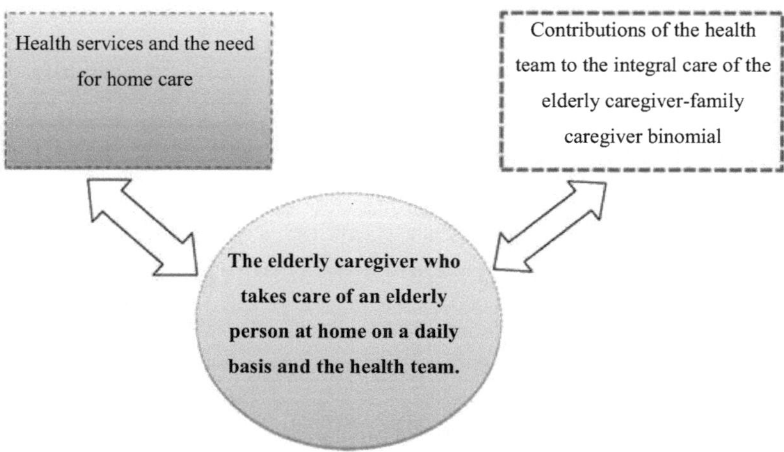

5.9.1 Health services and the need for home care

In this study, as has already been explained, the family caregiver is elderly and has compromised health and, in other cases, the frailty is due to the aging process; in addition, in this research, the caregiver is also elderly and dependent. It happens that the caregiver depends on other people to take turns providing care, in order to facilitate their daily routine.

Dependency on home care is becoming a serious public health problem in the country. This is due to the accelerated **aging process and the emergence of pathologies,** making it necessary to provide adequate conditions, such as infrastructure and support, for family caregivers to carry out their role of caring for dependent elderly people properly.

Look, I started looking after her because I lived with her, then the diabetes happened and she lost her left limb, her left leg, right? (Gedeao)

Well, I started looking after him when he had a stroke, in 96, my daughter, he got very bad, he was in the "public hospital" for many months. (Ruth)

Well, she has a pressure problem, she understands osteoporosis, she has to be very careful with osteoporosis, so she doesn't fall. (Isabel)

Well, she has a pressure problem, she went to the cardiologist who said that her jugulars are very clogged, he doesn't know how she can be like this, he explained it like this: it's like a torrent of rain stuck, it doesn't know where it's going, that's more or less how he put it, understand? In fact everything started to get complicated in 96, when she had a stroke, then a year later she had a seizure, the doctor said that after the stroke, she had to be taking phenobarbital[R] , as she wasn't, she had a seizure. Well, now that she's with me she's had two heart attacks, and now the doctor says she has early Alzheimer's, but every now and then she changes, she gets a bit weird, then she starts repeating everything, asking and repeating. (Dina)

Faced with the reality experienced by elderly caregivers in their homes, Primary Health Care, through the Family Health Strategy (ESF), now plays an essential role in health care, acting as a support for elderly family caregivers and the elderly relatives they care for, mainly because it is currently defined as the preferred gateway to the health system, based on the Home Care Service.

However, what can be seen from the data in this study is a **deficit in meeting the health needs of the elderly caregiver and dependent elderly binomial**, on the part of those who seek care in the network services, UAPS and the ESF team (consultations and, above all, home visits). Unfortunately, the care provided does not meet the health needs of the elderly and the users who need it do not have the family health team as a reference. In the study in question, the interviewees did not know how to identify the multi-professional team and generally only recognized the community health worker.

I don't get anything from anyone, nothing, except for the health agent, who comes, but says that our area doesn't have a doctor. Even so, "N" got up early one day and went to get the prescription for the tranquilizer we use, because without a prescription you can't buy the medicine and in this confusion she lost my SUS card, because it was a paper card, it was like this: she went to make the SUS cards, she put my name wrong, because that's Adameire...Then they went to fix it, but they haven't brought it back yet, it's another paper one, I kept using it, then she took it to get the prescription, she stayed there for a while, about three days, rolling it up, rolling it up, then she said she could get the prescriptions, but it's all very difficult. (Adameire)

Only the private doctor, because with SUS it's very difficult, even to get an appointment, I tried, but I spent a year trying to get an appointment with an endocrinologist and I couldn't get one. So, thank God, he gave us better conditions, we don't pay rent, so it's for us to pay for a consultation, exams, medication, right? It's for us to look after ourselves, isn't it? (Eunice)

The nurse's process of caring for the elderly caregiver and the dependent elderly, based on the Nursing Process, enables care based on Dorothea Orem's theoretical framework of self-care. From this perspective, in the support-education system proposed by the theory, nurses have the role of promoting the client as an active agent of self-care, encouraging decision-making, behavior control and the acquisition of knowledge and skills (OREM, 1995).

If the Family Health Teams are unable to carry out their role, because they end up meeting the spontaneous demands of the unit, what is happening is that the burden of care is passed on to the family, without proper support, often leaving the elderly caregiver in charge, with insipid home care and sporadic actions by the health team. This creates serious problems for the elderly family caregiver, who takes on the care without proper monitoring and training, which can lead to damage to the health of the person being cared for. The caregivers, in turn, have no way of going to the unit and end up self-medicating, among other actions that could be avoided. This situation of **care-seeking strategies/need for home care** can be seen in the following excerpts:

No, no one comes here, we don't have contact with anyone. (Ruth)

I just have a cough, but my son gave me some syrup and I'm much better now. (Dina)

Look, "C" is the only one, right? (referring to the CHA), she'*s* always here. The nurse, even last month [I asked her at this point if she knew the name of the nurse responsible for the area and she replied] "E", right? The one who gives injections [she was actually referring to the nursing technician]. Well, she injected my mother every month. Last month I called, I was tired of calling, asking, they didn't come to give my mother the injection. (Lia)

Because for him the doctor has to come here, he has no patience, he gets there and fights, everyone passes in front of him, I want to leave, I want to pee, I want to drink coffee, he gets nervous. He doesn't like going out, he gets sick if you take him out. (Joshua)

When I lived in "VE", the staff from the health center always came, visited, but here, we've been living here for two and a half years, and apart from the CHA, no one has ever come. Apart from her, no one has ever come, no doctor, no nurse, the letter that comes from HIPERDIA, I give it to them, just for them to keep, because they've never done a single visit here. After I moved here, they never followed up, neither for her nor for me. There they would take her blood at home when she needed it, which helped me a lot. We also went a long time without a doctor, right?

Just like there's medicine at the clinic, I know there is, but I can't get it, I end up having to buy it, if only someone who came to visit could bring it, it would help me a lot. We need it." (Talita)

This study made it possible to see what the family's search for health services is like and to identify the essential need to restructure home care services to meet the demands of the elderly and their caregivers. The home care service linked to the ESF is distinguished by the fact that it is a modality that encompasses health prevention and promotion actions in their entirety and includes the practice of health, social and economic policies, directly influencing the community's health-disease process.

The aim of home care is to overcome the institutional barriers to health care and is a new way of working for professionals, as it is inserted where all the individual's relationships take place, within the family and in the community, allowing professionals to work with real and effective possibilities, based on a comprehensive view of the context of each individual's and family's life.

However, the issue of effectively carrying out home care, in the specific case of this study, ADI, as advocated by current legislation, comes up. It can be seen that the professionals in the teams, especially the nurses, carry out numerous activities which, taken together, make up the totality of their actions. These include meeting the daily demand in the UAPS; the numerous actions aimed at covering the area per team; coordinating the ACS; the health programs that must be carried out, such as: women's and men's health; hypertensive/diabetic patients; immunization, with its campaigns and coverage targets to be achieved; educational actions; and also, compliance with planning by the professionals.

On this journey, home care, when it takes place, is done in a fragmented way, with a view to solving problems, preventing a comprehensive view of the process and, therefore, with low resolutiveness. In home care, the care is long term and is not just about treating and curing the disease, but about attending to the various situations that may arise in the family context, specifically in the study focused on the elderly binomial.

The search for **care** for the **health needs of dependent elderly people is** made up of the paths taken by family members in search of the health services available in the municipality where the research was carried out. These paths include the services of the different levels of health care (primary, secondary and tertiary), both public and private, as can be seen in the following statements:

So, the blood glucose and the thing the nurses at HIPERDIA taught me, the other things, taking care of people, when I was young I took care of children, so I already had my wits about me, so it was easy for me to adapt to the new life that God has given me. (Gedeao)

Until she didn't need serious treatment at the HU, but she is treated at the HU, just yesterday we went to the Rheumatologist, then when it was in May last year, we discovered that she had osteoporosis, until then we didn't know, she fell and fractured her pelvis, then she had to rest, then when she took the plate, the doctor said: you have to go to a Rheumatologist immediately because she has a lot of osteoporosis. (Isabel)

Accessibility is defined as the result of the relationship between the effective availability of health services and individuals' access to these services (FRENK, 1992). The issues of **accessibility and poor support from the public authorities** were mentioned by the interviewees in an outburst, especially in the case of Gedeao, whose wife is in a wheelchair because she has had her lower left limb amputated due to diabetes and is 74 years old. He routinely experiences situations that could be avoided if he looked at the accessibility rights of people with special needs and also with regular home care, as provided for by law.

We can't find any facilities. Especially what the government says, because there are no sidewalks for wheelchair users, there are no ramps. Then you get to a place that says it's preferential, you're going to stay right there, you have to stay 3, 4 hours, there are people who have to stay right there, who are sick, but have two arms, two legs, they're often still young, 25, 30 years old, but I mean, if you're in line, we have to respect it and stay too. (Gedeao)

And another place on [...] I have to get off at the [...] bus stop and walk down the hill pushing a chair, because there I've already asked, I've already spoken to politicians, I've already appealed, we've already signed a petition, there with the people who go to [...], for them to put a bus stop there, at least on the way down, to get out of there we have to walk down holding a chair all the way to [...]....] and on the way up it's more difficult, but if they put up a crosswalk the drivers have to respect it so we can cross, when it's raining we have to walk in the rain to get there [...] (Gedeao)

People with disabilities are the most exposed to comorbidities associated with their disability, which can lead to a greater need to use health services to maintain their physical and mental integrity. In the context of meeting these needs and services, there is the issue of accessibility to services which, if not appropriate, could result in disabled people facing obstacles that make it impossible for them to access health services.

From Eunice's point of view, her concern extends to people with financial difficulties because, as she said and as could also be seen during the interview, she has a good financial situation and is able to afford consultations, exams and medication that are not offered by the SUS, not to mention that she has a car and drives, which makes it easier for her to get around and, consequently, the care process. But, on the other hand, a large number of Brazilians don't have the same conditions, depend on the SUS and end up having to wait for months to get certain exams and other procedures, such as specific treatments and surgical procedures.

I'm retired, I worked a lot, I was the head of clothing. He's also retired, a lawyer for the railroad network, he worked a lot, he wrote a lot, look in the library, there are over three thousand books, I'll show you later. He was a writer, a journalist, he had a very active life. Now I'm worried about those who can't afford it, right? Because he takes very expensive medicines, the SUS gives the basics, for hypertension, diabetes, but most people have to buy them. (Eunice)

5.9.2 Contributions of the health team to the integral care of the elderly caregiver-elderly family member binomial

With the demographic and epidemiological profile of the Brazilian population changing, health education has become essential and should be seen as a dimension of the care process by health professionals. In this context, nurses stand out, above all because of their direct contact with the population, including guidance on risk behaviors, in order to promote health and prevent chronic non-communicable diseases. Thus, health professionals should act to guide the care of family caregivers in order to minimize the degree of dependence, which tends to increase the morbidity and mortality of the population.

It is important to emphasize that health education should be developed in all areas of health care. However, primary care, which is considered the preferred gateway to SUS care, should take place in the health unit and, when this is not possible, it should take place in the home, through home visits, where there is the opportunity to closely monitor the care provided, as well as daily life.

According to Santos (2014), as nurses are professionals who have care as the object of their work process, they must seek to establish a unique relationship with each user, family and community throughout their professional practice, which is essential to health education processes. It should be remembered that their field of competence includes health education, with a view to the shared construction of knowledge, whether for self-care, health promotion or the prevention of diseases and/or illnesses.

Interpersonal relationships develop as a result of the process of interaction. There are no unilateral processes in human interaction, because everything that happens in interpersonal relationships stems from two sources which, in this study, are the health professional and the caregiver. This research showed **the importance of active listening for the elderly:** how the participants feel valued and relieved by active listening, which helps caregivers create bonds with the health professional and feel comfortable expressing a wide range of feelings.

No one has ever been interested in my life like this. (Adameire)

I'd really like to thank you for coming, for listening to me, gee! No one has ever stopped to listen to me, to apologize if I've said things that won't even help you, if you want to come back, you'll always be very welcome. (Dina)

It's very difficult, when my daughter comes here, we want to talk, but she has a problem with tablets, cell phones, and calls one and calls another, so we talk a bit, listening is very good, but God gives strength.

It was very good, because I exposed my problem. We just put it away." (Eunice)

It's the first time anyone has listened to me. Thank God, when we talk to someone, we feel renewed, like this conversation we're having this morning, I won't forget it any time soon, because it's been healthy for me, it must be for you too. It's always good to talk, people who listen help us solve problems. (Gedeao)

This highlights the importance of therapeutic listening, the dialog process and adapting language when caring for the elderly. Seeking out the person of the caregiver, understanding their social context, their life habits, their possibilities for support and their support within the social network is essential for effective care at home.

Home visits are necessary as they allow health professionals to immerse themselves in the socio-cultural context of each elderly person under their care and thus guarantee quality care by allowing the use of strategies within the reality of the elderly person that facilitate therapeutic care in the home, as well as enabling the emergence of a link between team and caregiver, with a view to developing interpersonal relationships in an effective way, with the aim of providing comprehensive care for the individual.

The presence of a health professional makes day-to-day life easier, as they help with learning activities, knowing how to deal with pathology, as a source of information and the promotion of qualified care for the person being cared for. Greater effectiveness comes from paying attention to the spiritual dimension, combined with the use of interpersonal relationships with a view to the integral care of the being.

It is noteworthy that, from the point of view of the individuals, their rights related to health are incipient, as they have a vision based on the treatment of the disease and do not demonstrate knowledge of assistance based on health prevention.

Well, the doctor always comes to visit her, checks her blood pressure, sees how she's doing, you know? [...] Every now and then she comes, [...] comes here, the health worker, so thank God everything is fine. [...] The staff at the health center are very nice, silly, the health center has been open for a year and a bit, not even two years.

Here's what I do, I do everything with her, so if she goes to the doctor and I'm in need, I go and see her too, the staff at the "M" health center, I was used to it. [...] As I've only been here a short time, I can't say much about the staff at the health center, except that I really liked the health agent, he's an excellent person, even though I met him the day before yesterday at the health center, and today, when he came, it was already moments that I realized I have someone to count on You saw him, he gave me his phone number, he said that if I need him, just call. Wow! We feel supported, don't we? The nurse, too, as I said, helped me a lot." (Dina)

When we need it, they help, right [...] When we need it, "P" [ACS] schedules an appointment for one of us. Yeah, because just by coming to look after him here, like when he has a blood test, the [nursing technician], I think it's "M", right? A short woman who works in the "SC", she's the one who comes to take the blood. That's a big help to me so I don't have to, because oh! We don't have a car, we have to rely on the bus to go out with him and we really can't [laughs, seems to remember an episode]. And not having a car makes it difficult for you to go out with an elderly person, doesn't it? [questioning me] To take him there, he gets angry. He's always been like that, he's never liked going out. (Joshua)

Based on the data, it can be seen that the participants have basic knowledge of the health-disease process and that self-care is seen in a rudimentary way. Some of the statements that emerged from the accounts of the elderly affected by chronic pathologies about their **knowledge of treatment stand** out:

I take Pressat, the stuff, I'll get it for you (he went to get it), I take Lorax, Lorazepan 2 mg, 01 tablet at night. (Adameire)

I take medicine for my blood pressure, which is well controlled. (Dina)

My glucose is high, it must be because I keep drinking water like crazy. Food, I eat very little, but the water is the same, he said [referring to the doctor who attended her at the emergency unit] that I can't eat sweets. (Lia)

I have high blood pressure, I take losartan, I use a pump, because I have allergic bronchitis, two types of pump, an antidepressant, I have gastritis, I have reflux, I have sinusitis, I have everything that has ITE (laughs humorously), I have everything that has ITE. I've had tendonitis, because I used to work a lot with repetitive seamstress work, from the age of 11 until I was in my fifties, so I got tendonitis. I do my work, but it's in stages. The day I wash clothes I can't stand the pain in my arm, because I hang the clothes on the clothesline, right![...] I take controlled medication for depression, I've had treatment, because I've given it to myself. I forgot, my head too... [pause], I forgot. What's wrong with my head? Rhythm,

dysrhythmia, I've had it! I had a lot of headaches. So the other day I had a CT scan, and he said [referring to the doctor] no, Mrs. Joshua, what you have is sequelae, what you have here is from what you had, but there's no need to worry. (Joshua)

I take medicine for rheumatism, I take medicine for blood pressure because I have blood pressure too. (Isabel)

The type of care provided through groups for the elderly works as a strategy for intervening with these people, since it provides a space for exchanging experiences related to therapeutic self-care and, at the same time, provides clarification on general issues related to ageing and its specific repercussions on care to be carried out at home. However, they report not being able to leave the house to go to the health unit. Thus, it can be understood that the elderly caregiver, in the process of aging, suffering from chronic illnesses and having the role of providing comprehensive care, sometimes alone at home, ends up being deprived of some activities outside the home, due to the difficulty of getting around, the lack of a companion for the family member they care for, which restricts their space and their social network.

In cases where it is possible to go to the unit, groups with the elderly should be planned and conducted by an interdisciplinary team, using group dynamics, dialogue, topics of interest to the participants, clear and simple language, so that the elderly can be part of the meeting and participate actively, contributing their experiences of life and critically reflecting on their process of health and illness, while at the same time interacting with the participants, which helps to ensure that, at least in these moments, they can have some kind of social interaction.

Another method that can be used is health education, through play in the FHS interface. One study describes play with the use of theater in the family health strategy, which proved to be a new way of educating in health, with pertinent themes. According to the demand raised, this dynamic promotes the integration and socialization of the participants, with the exchange of experiences and the raising of problems common to the group. Through the performing arts, it is possible to break the monotony and silence, which leads to interactivity (SOARES; SILVA, L.; SILVA, P., 2011). If used with elderly caregivers, there will be a positive balance, since in old age, people feel more lonely, need to communicate, interact, in short, be listened to attentively. At the same time, with this practice, the elderly could share pleasant moments and relax from the tension they experience.

The participation of the elderly in training or support groups needs to be encouraged by health professionals, since they function as a space that enables the sharing of experiences related to care, the exchange of positive or negative experiences and the possibility of overcoming difficulties and negative feelings, such as anxieties, fears, insecurities, conflicts and tensions. On the other hand, for those who are unable to travel to the unit, home-based training should be planned, with a subsequent assessment of the knowledge acquired and the possibility of carrying out certain types of care without the accompaniment of a professional.

According to Silva *et al.* (2014), contact with families allows them to closely monitor the reality and progress of each elderly person and their family member. At each visit it is possible to get to know the family routine, their habits and beliefs, which is essential for choosing actions and their subsequent adherence to the changes. It is also worth noting that the team becomes recognized and taken as a reference.

In the home setting, the health team, including nurses, has a key role to play in helping caregivers to learn about the importance of self-care, as well as to assess the real possibility of providing care in an integral and solitary way. In addition, teaching them about their responsibilities in terms of care; knowing how to stimulate the self-care of the family member they are looking after, who often overburdens caregivers to carry out activities that could be done by the person themselves, but they don't do it out of fear and insecurity. And also by identifying when other support options need to be considered, such as the Home Care Service - SAD in another modality or encouraging other family members to take part in the process of caring for the dependent elderly person.

In this sense, the nurse's work in the home or in the health unit, together with the other professionals in the team, in the search for interaction between all areas, in order to resolve health situations, will promote an adaptation to better meet the needs of the elderly caregiver and their family.

Based on the above, the codification emerged: **accompanied by the ESF team** which, in the view of the elderly, would be the way in which the presence of the health professional can make their day-to-day lives easier, as it helps them learn activities and how to deal with the pathology, and also serves as a source of information, as well as guaranteeing better attention to being cared for:

Here's what I do, I do everything with her, so if she goes to the doctor and I'm in need, I go and see her too, the people at the clinic are used to it. (Dina)

After more than 20 years of implementation, with significant adherence to the family health strategy by Brazilian municipalities, we can see that, in practice, there has been greater coverage of the population. However, the inclusion of the type I Home Care modality in the context of the ESF is still being worked on in an incipient way by the teams. It is considered that this has been implemented in family health slowly, with difficulties for professionals, due to: the structure offered for its operation; professional training; and the lack of a professional profile to work in PHC. The implication of this has been, with exceptions, the composition of disconnected and inefficient multi-professional teams.

For the ESF to develop a process of building new practices, it is essential that the professionals involved articulate an integrated, interdisciplinary dimension, a relationship of knowledge and articulation of a "field of care production" common to all for the development of teamwork. It is necessary to incorporate not only new knowledge, but also a paradigm shift in the commitment to public management, which guarantees a practice based on the principles of health promotion.

In turn, management has a responsibility to rethink the way the ESF has been run, based on tedious programs, without taking a differentiated view of the distinct Brazilian reality. This often ends up imposing a work overload on the professional, who is unable to plan care in order to "meet" targets and coverage, which is not always the local reality. In addition to resizing staff, it is necessary to increase the number of human resources to work regularly in homes, in view of the issue addressed, the occurrence of a progressive aging process, which leads to an increase in the demand for home care services and, therefore, the number of professionals per team should be rethought, or the number of people cared for by the team should be reduced.

The elderly caregiver, without prior training, needs to receive guidance on how to proceed in everyday situations of caring for another person, on treatment, as well as on the process that led to their relative's dependency, in addition to the need to share doubts and other questions with the health professional. The positive or negative consequences of caring for an elderly person at home will depend on who is doing the caring and how well trained the family member is.

Therefore, periodic home visits by the health team are essential and necessary, so that during the visits the professionals are aware of the social and economic changes that affect family structures and, consequently, the position and role of the caregiver.

The scientific literature shows that the task of caring for dependent elderly people at home can have adverse effects, causing negative impacts and physical, emotional, social and financial overload. There is therefore a need to develop programs aimed at preventing these effects and working to improve the caregiver's quality of life. What about when the caregiver is also elderly? But what would be the best way to approach these caregivers? After a review, the studies are based on courses and training for caregivers, in UAPS and specialized centers, that is, outside the home, which can make it difficult for the caregiver to participate. Another point is that we didn't find many studies on family caregivers in old age in the literature. There is a lot about formal or informal caregivers, but without the emphasis on elderly family caregivers.

The health professional will be able to assess the elderly person's support network and maintain home monitoring to assess care, as well as offering appropriate support. According to the results of this literature review, the importance of the family is ensured by the fact that, when they take on care, they do not do so alone, but with the help of a network of spontaneous social relationships and mobilizing resources that go beyond the immediate circumstances, serving as support in times of need.

need and crisis. The network is therefore considered to be a fundamental resource and the main source of help, especially for families in need (GUTIERREZ & MINAYO, 2010).

The data obtained showed that home care makes a significant contribution to the care of both the elderly caregiver and the elderly family member being cared for. In this context, it is necessary to create a profitable strategy for society and the state, which can be done through: the professionals' knowledge of the reality experienced by the family; the likelihood of comprehensive and holistic care; as well as a reduction in care costs, due to a lower rate of hospitalization and early discharge. In short, Home Care with a Gerontological Approach provides a different kind of treatment for the patient, their caregiver and, finally, their family.

An initial step towards a professional approach with a global view of the person will be through interpersonal relationships, based on genuine active listening. Next, for the health professional to be able to access the client's spirituality/religiosity, it is essential to have a bond of trust, as well as the right time to broach the subject, using common sense. This approach can take place during the anamnesis, in a very natural way and, although there is no "ready-made recipe" for the spiritual approach, the moment when the patient himself brings up the issue, demonstrating the importance it plays in his life, is considered an excellent opportunity.

On the other hand, various tools have been created to facilitate the approach to spirituality for health professionals who wish to do so, but they still find it difficult to deal with the subject. These tools will serve as facilitators of the process, helping to obtain a spiritual history. It is important to note that some instruments can be applied in a few minutes, when lack of time is a problem, as in the case of the FICA Questionnaire, shown in Table 6 (PUCHALSKIC; ROMER, 2000).

If the elderly person reports not being religious, the health professional should direct their questions to: how the patient copes with the disease; what gives meaning and purpose to their life; and what cultural beliefs may have an impact on their treatment (KOENIG, 2005).

Chart 6 Instrument for accessing the spiritual dimension

FICA Questionnaire

F - Faith / belief

- Do you consider yourself religious or spiritual?

- Do you have spiritual or religious beliefs that help you deal with problems?

- If not: what gives you meaning in life?

I - Importance or influence

- What importance do you attach to faith or religious beliefs in your life?

- Have faith or beliefs ever influenced you in dealing with stress or health problems?

- Do you have any specific beliefs that could affect medical decisions or your treatment?

C - Community

- Are you part of a religious or spiritual community?

- How does she support you?

- Is there a group of people that you "really" love or that is important to you?

- Are communities such as churches, temples, centers, support groups important sources of support?

A - Action in treatment

- How would you like your doctor or health professional to consider the issue of religiosity / spirituality in your treatment?

- Indicate, refer to some spiritual / religious leader.

Source: PUCHALSKIC; ROMER, 2000. Taking a spiritual history allows clinicians to understand patients more fully.

6. CONNECTIONS AND INTERCONNECTIONS FOR THE APPROXIMATION OF A THEORETICAL MODEL FOR THE INTEGRAL CARE OF THE BINOMOUS: ELDERLY FAMILY CAREGIVER AND ELDERLY FAMILY CAREGIVER IN PRIMARY HEALTH CARE

I'll do my best to carry on, and God will do the impossible for me.

Claudiney Ribeiro

Based on the categories identified and the theoretical relationships established between them, it was possible to develop an analytical and explanatory process of the actions and interactions that made up the process of caring for an elderly person by an elderly family caregiver, which was represented by the central category: "the spiritual dimension influencing the life and care process of the elderly family caregiver", in the daily routine of care at home. This process is made up of three other sub-processes, which represent the symbolic meaning of the experience for the family caregiver. Each sub-process identified was named to form the respective categories: "growing old and becoming a caregiver", "family support" and "elderly caregiver who cares for an elderly person at home on a daily basis and the healthcare team".

From there, the problematic situation was identified and it was proposed to plan a strategy aimed at comprehensive care for the binomial, through Primary Health Care, at the interface of the Home Care Policy. The integration between the categories and their articulation with the central category allowed for the construction of connections and interconnections (Diagram 6), which represents a comprehensive care model for the elderly family caregiver and the elderly family member they care for.

DIAGRAM 6 - CONNECTIONS AND INTERCONNECTIONS FOR APPROACHING A THEORETICAL MODEL OF COMPREHENSIVE CARE FOR THE BINOMIAL: ELDERLY FAMILY CAREGIVER AND ELDERLY FAMILY CARED FOR IN PRIMARY HEALTH CARE

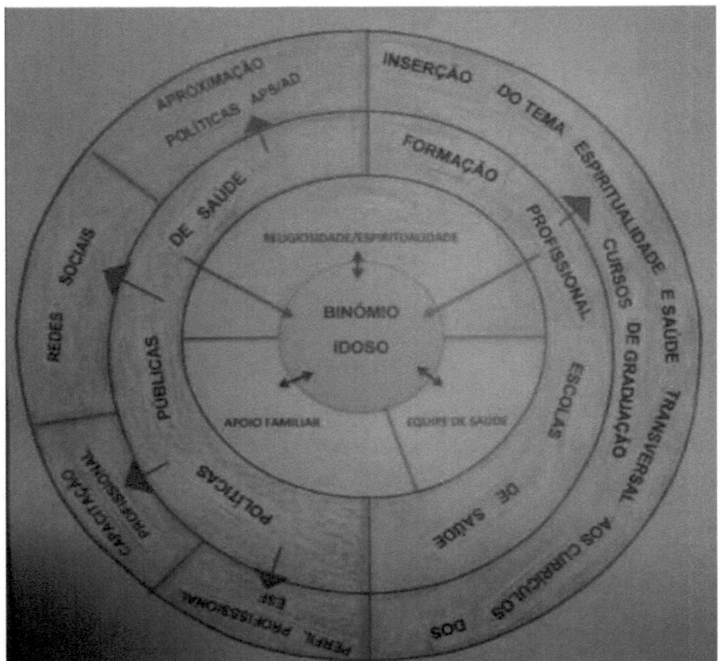

The study led to the realization that, for elderly family caregivers, what drives them, what keeps them going and makes them continue on the path of caring fully for another elderly person, regardless of what may happen or the family support they find to continue caring, is their belief in a transcendent being who, in the opinion of the caregivers who took part in the research, is God. Hence the strength they have is God's strength. According to the data analyzed, care is their responsibility 24 hours a day, seven days a week, and in this study, some caregivers reported having partial family support and others no family support at all.

For the elderly family caregiver, self-care does not exist unless it is combined with care for others, which allowed us to treat them as a pair. However, he tries to take care of himself and shows concern for his health, mainly because of the responsibility that coexists when, for him, someone depends on him to continue living.

As for the institutionalized care they receive, it is still incipient, irregular and unattended by the team as a whole, always fragmented, having been carried out by one or at most two members of the Family Health Team, sporadically and occasionally for the elderly person they care for. As a result, it is clear that the caregiver was unable to identify or classify the professionals in the health team; in some cases, they were able to identify the community health worker.

In order to understand the connections established, it is necessary to go back to what brought us here. This discussion has come about because of the demographic and epidemiological transition, which is leading to a rapid aging process and, as a result, we have to emphasize the role of the caregiver, who is becoming more important every day, especially the family caregiver and, above all, to study the elderly family caregiver, who is appearing on the scene with overwhelming frequency.

We will start from the premise that if we have a caregiver and someone depends on them, then it is necessary to provide comprehensive care for this individual who has set out to care for the other person in their entirety. Current policies are based on reducing hospitalization time, believing that it is better for the elderly to return home quickly. However, they forget that the focus of care should be on the family, in the specific case of this study, the couple. Considering that it is hoped that the elderly person who has some kind of dependency will not need successive hospitalizations, it is essential that the caregiver is healthy enough to continue caring.

In the case of the elderly caregiver, the subject of this study, more than a simple consultation to get a prescription, they have shown that they genuinely need to be listened to. The elderly caregiver wants to be listened to and to share their experiences, which are not easy; they need to speak, to know that they are being listened to, without judgment, without prejudice, but simply being listened to by someone who considers them important, because they are carrying out the noble task of caring for others and who, in order to do so, have given up their children, family, job and even their personal freedom. And the data showed us that they don't have the opportunity to be listened to by family members, professionals or other people.

It emerged from the data collected and the analysis carried out above that the process of caring is really a family one. The family is responsible, but then who will be responsible for the day-to-day care? After internal arrangements, the family caregiver emerges and then it will be necessary to take care of this new nuance. But how? First of all, the family health team needs to reconfigure the care it provides, since the elderly require a different look. The team also needs to access the spiritual dimension, which, for the elderly, was shown to be the most important category.

This study creates a number of possible nuances for primary health care through the multi-professional team. It starts with the new perspective that the team must take when dealing with the elderly in their area of work. Accessing the spiritual dimension, promoting effective interpersonal relationships, with a view to providing comprehensive care for the couple, involving them in their self-care and also encouraging them through guidance so that the cared-for family member exercises their own self-care, when possible, since the carer, out of insecurity, ends up taking on care for themselves that the other could be carrying out. There is no way to visit a home where the family lives with an elderly family caregiver without looking at the binomial, which until now has been forgotten. The professional who provides care in the home only looks at the elderly person being cared for, and their caregiver, as we saw in the study, has at least one chronic illness, in addition to the various factors that affect their mental health. In addition to having difficulties leaving the home, they also have to move away from the person they are caring for. Therefore, there is no denying the existence of the "caregiver" as part of the home care process.

On the other hand, faced with this serious public health problem, due to the sudden and progressive increase in the number of elderly people and the lack of preparation for this fact, there is an urgent need to restructure policies aimed at caring for the elderly; as well as creating and strengthening existing support networks; resizing teams, in view of the priority for home care; and, above all, attracting human resources with a profile for primary care. In addition, professionals who already work on the front line need to be trained to deal with the new demand: the elderly and spirituality and health.

On the other hand, as in the case of other countries, such as the United States, it is important to include subjects that include Spirituality in Health in professional training, because what we see today is the situation of health professionals who consider themselves unprepared to access the spiritual dimension when it comes to client care.

7. LIMITATIONS OF THE STUDY AND QUESTIONS FOR FUTURE RESEARCH

Get used to listening to the voice of your heart.

It is through him that God speaks to us and gives us the strength we need to move forward, overcoming the obstacles that come our way.

Sister Dulce

We know that, in a master's degree study, it is always possible for there to be flaws in the preparation, because time is short, and it becomes necessary to adopt a path to try to resolve the initial concerns that led to its execution. Some of the limitations of this study are outlined below.

A first point that stands out was the difficulty of going to the field and finding the research subjects, because there is no control of the total number of elderly family caregivers in the ESF areas, leading us to depend on the knowledge of the ACS. This could lead to another bias in the study, mainly due to the fact that there were no participants who presented a stance in opposition to care, i.e. neglect of the family member.

Another question is that the study did not find any non-religious caregivers with negative religious *coping,* nor any caregivers who showed opposition to the care of others. Could this be due to age? The researcher's impression of the participants was one of sincerity and concern for the other during the interviews and observations; however, the meetings were occasional.

The results allow us to understand the local situation of family caregivers of the elderly in the context of primary care, and the results can only be applied to groups similar to those used in this study. Another limitation was the small number of men in the study, which may influence the gender ratio.

It is therefore suggested that further research be carried out: longitudinal studies, with the same focus on primary care, and in other locations, in secondary and tertiary care, in order to make it possible to compare the information and expand the possibilities of care for elderly family caregivers and the elderly family member they care for.

8. FINAL CONSIDERATIONS

I'm grateful for all the difficulties I've faced; if it hadn't been for them, I wouldn't have gotten anywhere. Easy things stop us walking. Even criticism helps us a lot

Chico Xavierx

From the first moment I set out to do this work, there was a constant concern that it might contribute to enriching care for the elderly family caregiver who looks after another elderly person at home.

By analyzing the data collected, it became possible to glimpse how the process of caring for the ageing elderly takes place at home and how the main family caregiver perceives it. And, in the process, to understand the implications for their life and health, based on the meanings they give to this experience. In order to do this, it was necessary to capture and then articulate the emotional manifestations they described in depth and which were sometimes established in a scenario with an accumulation of daily tasks, which leads to an overload and emotional discomfort, as well as the fear of worsening of the clinical condition of the person being cared for and the lack of time, arising from the activities carried out by the caregiver and the difficulty in moving away from the person being cared for due to the bond of trust that is created between them.

Growing old and becoming a family caregiver is an activity that brings changes to people's lifestyles and is learned in the day-to-day lives of families, without prior preparation or training. Thus, through the home visits to the ten families involved in the research, it was possible to see that the choice of caregiver was based on need, due to compromised health conditions and the progressive decline in the caregiver's ability to take care of themselves, making them dependent on a full-time caregiver, which determined internal movements in the family structure, involving or distancing its members and resulting in the definition or self-designation of the member who would take on the role of family caregiver.

The study allowed us to understand the importance of family support for the elderly caregiver and the family member being cared for. The elderly family caregiver's life context is marked by interactions with close people: family and friends. Their influence on the situation was clear from the data. Sometimes in a positive way, serving as support and encouragement; at other times, in opposition, the lack of support has a negative influence on the whole process of caring for others, including the caregiver's health. Elderly family caregivers who look after dependent elderly people dedicate themselves fully and, most of the time, without the help of other family members in the division of tasks, and this direct exposure, over time, contributes to a greater risk of illness, deficits in self-care, increased burden and emotional discomfort.

The results of this research have enabled us to understand the process of caring for elderly family caregivers who look after other elderly people at home. By getting to know the daily lives of elderly caregivers, I was able to observe positive and negative aspects and repercussions that directly or indirectly influence their health, as well as the process of caring for others. It is clear that health professionals, especially nurses, can help to improve the quality of life of the couple by training caregivers. It was possible to identify that, in the subjects' understanding, their experiences in the face of the reality of their lives, with the arduous task of fully caring for the other at home, without prior preparation, specific demands for support for the caregiver appear, which will favor the process of adapting to caring for the other, who will have greater security in carrying out the care. In addition, better organization of time, as well as the prioritization of tasks and, thus, the gaining of time to carry out self-care in a comprehensive way, that is, with the aim of maintaining life, health and well-being.

Family health teams need to integrate the concepts of interdisciplinarity and set up a family support-education system, helping in the planning and execution of care. Through the interpersonal relationship between the family health team and between the family and the caregiver, based on a new view of the elderly caregiver, who shows genuine interest in someone who listens to them and is interested in their life story.

However, even in the face of the negative repercussions and difficulties experienced by the elderly family caregiver, and regardless of whether or not they have the support of family or are institutionalized, they are empowered to face the daily challenges of being a family caregiver by the spiritual dimension. At this stage of life, there is a change in perspective from a materialistic and pragmatic view of the world to a more cosmic and transcendent view.

While they seek support from a metaphysical force, the participants use spiritual religious *coping,* which are the strategies they use to deal with situations that may arise in their lives and attribute to the sacred the strength to persevere and continue on their path, growing old and caring for one or more elderly people at home.

Health professionals must remain alert to the needs related to the spiritual dimension of the elderly and be sensitized to this aspect in the search for health care, based on a humanistic view of the human being. It is therefore necessary to access the spiritual dimension as an auxiliary element in the process of health care for the elderly, given that spirituality is heightened at this stage of life.

It is hoped that this research will contribute to giving visibility to home care in the context of health policies. It is also hoped that the study will provide support for the process of care provided by family health teams that care for elderly people and contribute to the redesign of professional actions for the health of elderly caregivers. Furthermore, by being aware of the difficulties and demands presented by these individuals in carrying out self-care and caring for others, nurses within this team can rethink the organization of the work process, evaluating health education activities such as support/training groups and carrying out regular home visits as a priority and with a comprehensive look at the family. In this way, we can help to reduce the tension experienced on a daily basis; access the spiritual dimension; promote effective interpersonal relationships, with a view to providing comprehensive care for the couple, involving them in their self-care; and encourage, through guidance, the caregiver to exercise self-care whenever possible.

It is believed that by disseminating the study, it will also be possible to contribute to building knowledge on the subject. On the other hand, health schools in general need to include subjects that address the theme of "spirituality and health" in the training of health professionals, with the aim of better preparing them to deal with such demands in their professional practice. This is because, in the current reality, professionals prefer to shy away from tackling the subject because they claim to be unprepared. The most effective way of ingraining values and attitudes of respect for human life is in the training process, where themes can be consolidated that will consolidate an innovative culture of health care.

9. REFERENCES

ALBERTONI, F.P. A acção dos sujeitos sociais na urbanizaçao da regiao de Sao Pedro em Juiz de Fora/MG. Juiz de Fora: Dissertation (academic master's degree) - Federal University of Juiz de Fora, School of Social Work. Postgraduate Program in Social Work, 95f. p 55, 2014.

ALLIANCE FOR AGING RESEARCH. Fact Sheet: Selected Caregiver Statistics. 2011.

ALMEIDA, S. T. G. et al. Care Of The Elderly: Factors That Influence The Performance Of Health Professionals In Primary Care. **Revista de Pesquisa: Cuidado é Fundamental Online**, n. Supl., p. 135-144, 2012.

ALLPORT, G.W. **The individual and his religion**. London: Macmillan, 1950.

ALVES, JED, BARROS, LFW, CAVENAGHI, S. The dynamics of religious affiliations in Brazil between 2000 and 2010: diversification and the process of changing hegemony. REVER (PUC-SP), v. 12, p. 145-174, 2012.

ALVES, L. C.; LEITE, I. C.; MACHADO, C. J. Conceptualizing and measuring functional disability in the elderly population: a literature review. **Ciênc Saùde Coletiva**, v. 13, n. 4, p. 1199-207, 2008.

ALVES, L. C.; LEITE, I. C.; MACHADO, C. J. Factors associated with functional disability among the elderly in Brazil: a multilevel analysis. **Rev Saùde Pùblica**, v. 44, n. 3, p. 468-78, 2010.

ARAÙJO, I. M. ; PAUL, C.; MARTINS, M. M. Caring for dependent elderly people at home: stories from caregivers - DOI: 10.4025/cienccuidsaude. v8i2. 8198. **Ciência, Cuidado e Saùde**, v. 8, n. 2, p. 191-197, 2009.

ARAÙJO, J. S. et al. The obligation to (un)care: social representations of care for stroke patients by their caregivers. **Revista Mineira de Enfermagem**, v. 16, n. 1, p. 98-105, 2012.

ASSOCIATION OF RELIGION DATA ARCHIVES, A. Measures. **The Pennsylvania State University**, 1998.

ATKINSON, L. D.; MURRAY, M. E. Nursing Practice: Fundamentals and Ethics. Atkinson, LD; Murray, ME. **Fundamentals of Nursing. Introduction to the nursing process.** Translated by Ademar Valadares Fonseca. Ed. Guanabara Koogan, p. 203-211, 1989.

BARBOSA, B. R. et al. Evaluation of the functional capacity of the elderly and factors associated with disability. **Centro**, v. 39, p. 002, 2014.

BARRA, S. A.R. **Gestao da Estratégia Saùde da Familia: o desafio de consolidar a intersetorialidade.** Dissertation (Master's Degree in Social Work) - School of Social Work, Federal University of Juiz de Fora, Juiz de Fora, 200f. p. 46, 2013.

BAUNGART, T.A.A.; AMATUZZI, M.M. "Religious Experience and Personal Growth: A Phenomenological Understanding". **Revista de Estudos da Religiao.** Sao Paulo, n°4: 95111, 2007.

BOCCHI, S. C. M.; ANGELO, M. Between freedom and confinement: social support as a component of the quality of life of the family caregiver-dependent person binomial. **Rev. Latino-Am. Enfermagem**, Ribeirao Preto , v. 16, n. 1, p. 15-23, Feb. 2008 .

BLUMER, H. **Symbolic Interactionism: Perspective and Method**. University of California Press. ISBN 9780520056763. 1986.

BOFF, L. Saber Cuidar: Ética do humano, Compaixao pela Terra. Petrópolis, R.J., Vozes, 1999.

BOFF, L. Spirituality. A path to transformation. Rio de Janeiro: Sextante, 2001, p. 66.

BOHM, V; CARLOS, S. A. **Caring for the elderly: feelings triggered by this relationship** *Revista Kairós Gerontologia, 13*(1), Sao Paulo, June 2010: 211-20.

BRAAM, A. W. et al. Cosmic transcendence and framework of meaning in life: Patterns among older adults in The Netherlands. **The Journals of Gerontology Series B: Psychological Sciences and Social Sciences**, v. 61, n. 3, p. S121-S128, 2006.

BRAZIL. Ministry of Health (BR). Portaria no. 2.528 de 19 de outubro de 2006a: Aprova a **Politica Nacional da Saùde da Pessoa Idosa**. Diàrio Oficial Repùblica Federativa do Brasil 2006a Oct; 237(20)4, , p.3.

. Ministry of Health (BR). Ordinance No. 971, of May 3, 2006. Provides for the National Policy for Integrative and Complementary Practices (PNPIC) in the Unified Health System. Official Journal of the Union 2006c.

. Ministry of Health. Law No. 10.741, of October 10, 2003, which provides for the Statute for the Elderly and makes other provisions. **Official Gazette of the Federative Republic of Brazil,** Brasilia (DF), 2003.

. Ministry of Health (MS). Ordinance No. 1.395/GM, of December 10, 1999. Approves the **National Elderly Health Policy**. Brasilia: MS; 1999.

. Secretariat of Health Care. **Manual for the Organization of Primary Care**. 4. ed. Brasilia, 1999a.

Ministry of Health. **Ordinance. 399/GM**, of February 22, 2006b.

. Ministry of Health. Secretariat of Science, Technology and Strategic Inputs. Department of Science and Technology. **Agenda nacional de prioridades de pesquisa em saùde**. 2. ed., Brasilia: Ministério da Saùde, 2008a.

. Ministry of Health (BR). Ordinance no. 2.488 of October 21, 2011: Approves the **National Primary Care Policy**, establishing revised guidelines and norms for the organization of Primary Care, for the Family Health Strategy (ESF) and the Community Health Agents Program (PACS). Diàrio Oficial Repùblica Federativa do Brasil. 2011a.

. Health Care   Secretariat. Ordinance No. 2527, of October 27, 2011. Redefines **Home Care within the scope of the Unified Health System**. Official Gazette of the Federative Republic of Brazil, Brasilia (DF), 28 Oct 2011b: Section 1:1.

. Health Care Secretariat. **Ordinance No. 963, of May 27, 2013**. Brasilia: Ministry of Health, 2013.

. Ministry of Health. Health Care Secretariat. Secretariat for Work Management and Health Education. **Practical guide for caregivers.** Brasilia: Ministry of Health, 2008b.

. Ministry of Health. National Health Council, National Committee for Ethics in Research on Human Beings. Resoluçao 466, de 12 de dezembro de 2012: **diretrizes e normas regulamentadoras de pesquisa envolvendo seres humanos.** Official Gazette of the Federative Republic of Brazil, Brasilia (DF), 2012.

. Constitution of the Federative Republic of Brazil. Brasilia: Senado Federal; Centro Gràfico. 1998.

. Ministry of Health. Institute for Health Development. **Nursing Manual: Family Health Program.** Brasilia: 2001.

. Ministry of Social Development and Fight against Hunger. National Policy for the Elderly. 1. ed. Brasilia, Reprinted 2010.

BRITO, M. J. M. et al. Home care in the structuring of the health care network: treading the paths of integrality. **Escola Anna Nery Revista de Enfermagem**, v. 17, n. 4, p. 603-610, 2013.

BUTLER, R. N. The longevity revolution: The benefits and challenges of living a long life. New York, NY: Public Affairs; 2008.

CABRAL, D. F. et al. Anxiety, stress and depression in family caregivers of the mentally ill.

Atencion Primaria, *46*, 176-179, 2014.

CAMARANO, A.A.; KANSO S.; PASINATO M.T.; MELLO J. L. E. Idosos brasileiros - indicadores de condiçoes de vida e de acompanhamento de politicas. Brasilia: Presidency of the Republic/Subsecretariat of Human Resources; 2005.

CAMARGO JUNIOR, K. R. de. **Introducing Logos**: a textual data manager. Institute of Social Medicine - UERJ, Rio de Janeiro, 2003. p.30.

CARREIRA, L.; RODRIGUES, R. A. P. Dificuldades dos familiares de idosos portadores de doenças crônicas no acesso à Unidade Bàsica de Saùde. **Rev Bras Enferm**, v. 63, n. 6, p. 933-9, 2010.

CARVALHO, M. C. B. (org.). Familia contemporànea em debate. Sao Paulo: Cortez, 2003.

CASADO, B; SACCO, P. Correlates of caregiver burden among family caregivers of older Korean Americans. **The Journals of Gerontology Series B: Psychological Sciences and Social Sciences**, v. 67, n. 3, p. 331-336, 2012.

CASTRO, E. A. B. Weaving the safety net after a fall: care after discharge. In: CAMARGO JUNIOR, K. R. **Por uma filosofia empirica da atença à saù**: olhares sobre o campo biomédico. Rio de Janeiro: Editora Fiocruz, 2009. p. 155-87.

CECILIO, L.C. O. Theoretical-conceptual notes on evaluation processes considering the multiple dimensions of health care management. **Interface (Botucatu)**, Botucatu , v. 15, n. 37, p. 589-599, June 2011 .

CELICH, K.L.S.; BATISTELLA, M. Being a family caregiver of Alzheimer's disease patients: unveiled experiences and feelings. **Cogitare Enferm.**, Rio Grande do Sul, v. 12, n. 2, Apr.-Jun., 2007.

CHAIMOWICZ, F. Health of the elderly / Flâvio Chaimowicz with the collaboration of: Eulita M. Barcelos, Maria D. S. Madureira and Marco Túlio de F. Ribeiro. - 2. ed. Belo Horizonte: NESCON/UFMG; 2013.

CHARMAZ, K. **The construction of grounded theory**: a practical guide to qualitative analysis. Porto Alegre: Artmed; 2009 p. 23-28.

COLLIÈRE, Marie-Françoise - *Promoting life: from the practice of women of virtue to nursing care.* Lisbon: Lidel, 1999. ISBN 972-757-109-3;

COMTE-SPONVILLE, A. *The Spirit of Atheism.* Sao Paulo: Martins Fontes, 2007.

CORBO, A. D.; MOROSINI, M. V. G. C. Family health: recent history of the reorganization of health care. In: Escola Politècnica de Saù Joaquim Venâncio (Org.). **Textos de apoio em politicas de saù**. Rio de Janeiro: Fiocruz, 2005. p. 157-181.

COSTA, A. C. A. S. Nurses and social representations of ageing: implications for autonomy-promoting care for hospitalized elderly people. 2011.

COSTA, S. R. D. ; C. E. A. B.; ACIOLI, S. Self-care capacity of hospitalized adults and elderly: implications for nursing care< sup>*</sup>. **Revista Mineira de Enfermagem**, v. 17, n. 1, p. 193-207, 2013.

COUTO, A. M. **Family caregiver of dependent elderly**: experiences of caring in the home context and implications for Nursing. 2013. Dissertation (Academic Master's Degree in Nursing)-Postgraduate Program in Nursing, Federal University of Juiz de Fora, Juiz de Fora, 177f. 2013.

DALGALARRONDO, P. **Religiao, psicopatologia e saù mental**. Porto Alegre: Artmed, 2008.

DE ALMA ATA, D. International Conference on Primary Health Care; September 6-12, 1978. **Alma Ata, USSR.**

DE CARVALHO DANTAS, C. et al. Data-based theory - conceptual and operational aspects: a possible methodology to be applied in nursing research. **Rev Latino Am Enfermagem**, v. 17, n. 4, 2009.

DE FREITAS, M. H. Religiosity and health: patients' experiences and professionals' perceptions. **Revista Pistis Praxis**, v. 6, n. 1, 2014.

DENZIN, N. K; LINCOLN, Y. S. **Hand-book of qualitative research**. Thousand Oaks: Sage, 1994. p.2.

DICK, B. Grounded Theory: a thumbnail sketch. 2005.

DIOGO, M. J.D. Nursing Consultation in Gerontology. In: Netto, Matheus Papaléo. Tratado de Gerontologia, 2.ª ed. Revised and expanded. Sao Paulo; Atheneu, 2007. p.377-392.

DYSON, J. COBB, M. The meaning of spirituality: a literature review. J Adv Nurs. 1997; 26(6); 1183-8.

ELIAS, N. A solidao dos moribundos followed by "Envelhecer e Morrer". Rio de Janeiro: Jorge Zahar 1985.

ELIOPOULOS, C. **Gerontological nursing**. 7. ed. Porto Alegre: Artmed, 2011.

ELSEN, I.; MARCON, S. S.; SILVA, M. R.S. (Org.). O viver em familia e sua interface com a saù e a doença. 2? ed. Maingà: Eduem, 2004. 460p.

ERDMANN, L. et al. Building a care system model. **Acta Paul Enferm**, v. 20, n. 2, p. 180-5, 2007.

ERIKSON J. The Gerotranscendence. In: Erikson E. **The life cycle completed: a review**. Extended version with new chapters from Joan M. Erikson. New York, NY: W. W. Norton & Company, Inc. 1998. p. 123-9.

FARAH, B. F. Continuing education in the process of organizing health services: the repercussions of the introductory course for Family Health teams-experience in the municipality of Juiz de Fora/MG. Rio de Janeiro: Institute of Social Medicine, Rio de Janeiro State University, 2006.

FERNANDES, M.G.M.; GARCIA, T.R. Attributes of stress in family caregivers of dependent elderly people. **Rev. esc. enferm. USP**, Sao Paulo, v. 43, n. 4, p. 818-24, 2009.

FERNANDES, M. T. O.; SOARES, S. M. O desenvolvimento de politicas pùblicas de atença ao idoso no Brasil.**Rev. esc. enferm. USP**, Sao Paulo , v. 46, n. 6, Dec. 2012.

FRAGOSO, S.; RECUERO, R.; AMARAL, A. Métodos de pesquisa para internet. Porto Alegre: Sulina, 2011.

FREITAS, R. S. et al. Functional capacity and associated factors in the elderly: a population-based study. **Acta Paul Enferm**, v. 25, n. 6, p. 933-939, 2012.

FRENK, J. et al. The concept and measurement of accessibility. In: **OPS. Scientific Publication**. Pan American Health Organization, 1992. p. 929-943.

FRIES, A. T.; PEREIRA, D. C. Theories of Human Aging. **Revista Contexto & Saùde**, v. 10, n. 20, p. 507-514, 2011. ISSN 2176-7114.

GAMLIEL, T. A Social Version of Gerotranscendence: Case Study. **Journal of Aging and Identity.** Vol. 6. N. 2, p. 105-114, 2001.

GASQUE, K. C. G. D. Grounded theory: a new perspective for exploratory research. In: MUELLER, Suzana Pinheiro Machado (Org.). Métodos para a pesquisa em Ciência da Informaçao. Brasilia: Thesaurus, 2007. p. 83-118.

GEERTZ, C. **The interpretation of cultures**. Rio de Janeiro: Ed. Zahar, 1978.

GIOVANETTI, J. P. Existential Psychology and Spirituality. In. AMATUZZI, M. M. (org.). Psychology and Spirituality. Sào Paulo, Ed. Paulus. 2005. p. 129 - 145.

GLASER, B. G.; STRAUSS, A. L. **The discovery of grounded theory**: strategies for qualitative research. New York: Aldine Publishing, 1967.

GOLDDTEIN, L. L.; SOMMERHALDER, C. Religiosity, spirituality and existential meaning in adulthood and old age. In: Freitas et al: Tratado de geriatria e gerontologia. Rio de Janeiro: Guanabara Koogan, 2002.

GOMES, K. O. et al . Atenção Primària à Saù - a "menina dos olhos" do SUS: sobre as representações sociais dos protagonistas do Sistema Ùnico de Saù. **Ciênc. saùde coletiva**, Rio de Janeiro , v. 16, supl. 1, 2011 .

GONZAGA, M. R. The future of the Brazilian population: methodological and operational aspects for population projections in Brazil. **Revista Coletiva**, N.13, Apr. 2014.

GUIMARÂES, M. B. A. Intuition in the clinic: building links between reason and emotion. In: VASCONCELOS, E. M. (org.). A espiritualidade no trabalho em Saúde. Sao Paulo, Editora Hucitec, 2006 p. 325-357.

GUNTER L.M.; MILLER J.C. Toward a nursing gerontology. Nurs. Res; 1977; 26: 208.

GUTIERREZ, D.M.D; MINAYO, M.C.S. (2010). Production of knowledge on health care within the family. *Ciência e Saùde Coletiva*, *15*(supl.1), 497-508.

HUFFORD, D. J. An Analysis of the Field of Spirituality, Religion and Health (S/RH). 2005.

IBGE. Ministry of Planning. **Population projection by sex and age: Brazil** 20002050. Brasilia: IBGE. 2013.

. Ministry of Planning. **Summary of Social Indicators -2009**. Brasilia: IBGE. 2009.

Ministry of Planning. **Synopsis of the demographic survey. Brazilian Institute of Geography and Statistics.** Brasilia: IBGE. 2010a.

. Ministry of Planning. Synopsis of the demographic survey. Brazilian Institute of Geography and Statistics. Brasilia: IBGE. **Distribution of the population by sex, according to age groups - Juiz de Fora.** 2010b.

. Ministry of Planning. Synopsis of the demographic survey. Brazilian Institute of Geography and Statistics. Brasilia: IBGE. **Distribution of the population by sex, according to age groups - Uberlândia.** 2010c.

. Ministry of Planning. Synopsis of the demographic survey. Brazilian Institute of Geography and Statistics. Brasilia: IBGE. **Distribution of the population by sex, according to age groups - Minas Gerais.** 2010d.

. Ministry of Planning. Synopsis of the demographic survey. Brazilian Institute of Geography and Statistics. Brasilia: IBGE. **Distribution of the population by sex, according to age groups - Brazil.** 2010e.

. Ministry of Planning. Synopsis of the demographic survey. Brazilian Institute of Geography and Statistics. Brasilia: IBGE. **2010 Demographic Census: General characteristics of the population, religion and people with disabilities.** Rio de Janeiro, 2012.

JARDIM, S.E.G. Aspectos socioeconômicos do Envelhecimento. In: Netto, Matheus Papaléo. Tratado de Gerontologia, 2.ª ed. Revised and expanded. Sao Paulo; Atheneu, 2007.

JUIZ DE FORA. Juiz de Fora City Hall. History of the City. 2014a.

. Juiz de Fora City Hall. Juiz de Fora Basic Sanitation Plan. 2014b.

. City Hall. Health Department. **Master Plan for Primary Health Care - Implementation Project.** Thiago Campos Horta, Maria Aparecida Martins Baêta

Guimaraes, Clàudia Rocha Franco, Ana Paula Brandao Costa. Juiz de Fora (MG), 2014c. 133p.

. **Municipal Health Plan. Annual Health Program**. Department of Health, Sanitation and Environmental Development - SSSDA, Juiz de Fora, 2014d.

JARDIM, S.E.G. Aspectos socioeconômicos do Envelhecimento. In: Netto, Matheus Papaléo. Tratado de Gerontologia, 2. ed. Revised and expanded. Sao Paulo; Atheneu, 2007.

KING, J. E.; CROWTHER, M. R. The measurement of religiosity and spirituality: Examples and issues from psychology. **Journal of Organizational Change Management**, v. 17, n. 1, p. 83-101, 2004.

KOENIG, H. G. Spirituality in patient care. Why, how, when and what. Sao Paulo: **Editora FE,** 2005.

KOENIG, H. G.; MCCULLOUG, M.; LARSON, D. B. **Handbook of religion and health:** a century of research reviewed. New York: Oxford University Press, 2001.

KOENIG, H. G. ; BÜSSING, A. The duke university religion index (DUREL): A five-item measure for use in epidemological studies. **Religions**, v. 1, n. 1, p. 78-85, 2010.

KOENIG, H. ; KING, D.; CARSON, V. B. **Handbook of religion and health.** 2.ed. 2012.Oxford University Press, 2012 p.37-38 .

KUBLER-ROSS, E. The wheel of life. Memories of living and dying. 2. ed. Sextante, 1998 p.13.

LAVELA, S. L. ; ATHER, N. Psychological health in older adult spousal caregivers of older

158

adults. **Chronic Illness**, v. 6, n. 1, p. 67-80, 2010.

LAVRAS, C. Primary health care and the organization of regional health care networks in Brazil. **Saùde e Sociedade**, v. 20, n. 4, p. 867-874, 2011.

LEME, L. E.G. The elderly and the family. In: Netto, Matheus Papaléo. Treatise on Gerontology, 2.ª ed. Revised and expanded. Sao Paulo; Atheneu, 2007. p.217-223.

LEVACOV, Marilia. Grounded Theory. 2003.

LIMA, T. J. V. D. et al. Humanization in Elderly Health Care. **Saude soc.**, Sao Paulo, v. 19, n. 4, Dec. 2010 .

LINDOLPHO, M. C.; SA, S. P. C.; ROBERS, L. M. V. Spirituality/Religiosity, a support in nursing care for the elderly. **In Extension**, v. 8, n. 1, 2009.

LOPES, R.G. C; CALDERONI, S.Z. **"The family educating for peace"**. The family and the elderly: The possibility of meeting. Sao Paulo: Marco Markovitch, 2002. p. 102.

LOPES, R.G. C; CALDERONI, S.Z. The elderly in the family: Expanding Possibilities or

Retraction? In: Netto, Matheus Papaléo. Tratado de Gerontologia, 2.ª ed. Revised and expanded. Sao Paulo; Atheneu, 2007. p.225-231.

LOTUFO NETO F. The Prevalence of Mental Disorders among Religious Ministers. Thesis presented to the Faculty of Medicine of the University of Sao Paulo for the title of Full Professor in the Department of Psychiatry Sao Paulo, 1997. p.1-11.

LUCCHETTI, G. et al. Spirituality in clinical practice: what clinicians should know. **Rev Bras Clin Med**, v. 8, n. 2, p. 154-8, 2010.

LUCCHETTI, G. et al. Religiousness affects mental health, pain and quality of life in older people in an outpatient rehabilitation setting. **Journal of Rehabilitation Medicine**, v. 43, n. 4, p. 316-322, 2011.

LUCCHETTI, G. et al. **Integrating Spirituality into Primary Care**. INTECH Open Access Publisher, 2012.

MACRAE, J.A. Nursing as a spiritual practice: acontemporary application of Florence Nightingale's views. New York (NY): Springer; 2001.

MANNING, L. K. Navigating Hardships in Old Age: Exploring the Relationship Between Spirituality and Resilience in Later Life. 2013. Qualitative Health Research, *23*(4), 568-575. doi:10.1177/1049732312471730

MANOEL, M.F. et al. Family relationships and the level of family caregiver burden. **Escola**

Anna Nery Revista de Enfermagem, v. 17, n. 2, p. 346-353, 2013.

MARCON, S. S. et al. Familias cuidadoras de pessoas com dependência: um estudo bibliogràfico. Online **Brazilian Journal of Nursing**, Rio de Janeiro, v. 6, n. 1, 2006.

MATTA, G. C. The world health organization: from epidemic control to the struggle for hegemony. Trabalho Educaçao e Saùde, 3(2) p. 371-396, 2005.

MAZZA, M. M. P. R.; LEFÈVRE, F. Family caregiving: analysis of the social representation of the relationship between the family caregiver and the elderly. **Revista brasileira de crescimento e desenvolvimento humano,** v. 15, n. 1, p. 1-10, 2005. ISSN 0104-1282.

MCGHAN, G. et al. "End-of-Life Caregiving: Challenges Faced by Older Adult Women". **Journal of gerontological nursing** 39.6,45-54. PMC, 2013.

MCSHERRY, W.; JAMIESON, S. An online survey of nurses' perceptions of spirituality and spiritual care.(Survey). **Journal of Clinical Nursin.** 20(11 12), 1757, 2011.

. The qualitative findings from an online survey investigating nurses' perceptions of spirituality and spiritual care. **Journal of Clinical Nursing**, 22: 3170-3182. doi: 10.1111/jocn.12411, 2013.

MINAYO, M. C. S. **O desafio do conhecimento**: pesquisa qualitativa em saùde. 12 ed. Sao Paulo: Hucitec, 2010.

MONOD, S. M. et al. The spiritual distress assessment tool: an instrument to assess spiritual distress in hospitalized elderly persons. 2010. **BMC Geriatrics,** *10,* 88. doi:10.1186/1471-2318-10-88.

MONTEIRO, D. M. Spirituality and Ageing. In: Py, L. et al. **Tempo de Envelhecer: percursos e dimensôes Psicossociais** - 2ª ed. Holambra, SP: Ed. Setembro, 2006.

MOREIRA-ALMEIDA, A. et al. Religious involvement and sociodemographic factors: results of a national survey in Brazil. **Rev Psiq Clin**, v. 37, n. 1, p. 12-5, 2010.

MOREIRA-ALMEIDA, A.; LOTUFO NETO, F.; KOENIG, H. G. Religiousness and mental health: a review. **Rev. Bras. Psiquiatr.**, Sao Paulo , v. 28, n. 3, Sept. 2006.

MÜLLER, W. **Letting yourself be touched by the sacred**. Petrópolis: Vozes, p.31, 2004.

NATIONAL CENTER OF COMPLEMENTARY AND ALTERNATIVE MEDICINE. What is complementary and alternative medicine? [Internet]. **Bethesda: NCCAM**; 2007.

NORTH AMERICAN NURSING DIAGNOSIS ASSOCIATION. NANDA. NANDA nursing diagnoses: definitions and classification 2009-2011. Porto Alegre: Artmed; 2010.

NARDI, F. R; OLIVEIRA, M. F.L. Knowing the social support to the family caregiver of the dependent elderly. **Revista Gaûcha de Enfermagem**, v. 29, n. 1, p. 47, 2008.

NIGHTINGALE, F. **Notas sobre enfermagem:** o que é e o que não é. Translated by Amâlia Correa de Carvalho. Sao Paulo: Cortez: ABEn-CEPEn, 1989.

WHO - United Nations Organization. **Global guide to age-friendly cities.** 2009. Version translated into Portuguese.

OREM, D. **Nursing concepts of practice**. 5.ed. New York: Mosby, 1995.

PANZINI, R. G. Religious-Spiritual Coping Scale (CRE Scale): translation, adaptation and validation of the RCOPE Scale, addressing relationships with health and quality of life. **Religious-Spiritual Coping Scale (CRE Scale): translation, adaptation and validation of the RCOPE Scale, addressing relationships with health and quality of life**, 2004.

PANZINE, R. G.; ROCHA, N. S.; BANDEIRA, D.R.; FLECK, M. P. A. Quality of life and spirituality. **Rev. Psiq. Clin**. N. 34, supl. 1, p. 105-115, 2007.

PANZINI R. G, BANDEIRA D. R. Religious/spiritual coping. **Rev Psiquiatr Clin** 2007; 34(1):26-135.

PANZINI R. G, BANDEIRA D.R. Religious-spiritual coping scale (cre scale): elaboration and construct validation. **Psicol Estud** 2005; 10(3): 507-516.

PARGAMENT, K. I.; ANO, G. Empirical advances in the psychology of religion and coping. **Religious influences on health and well-being in the elderly**, p. 114-140, 2004.

PARGAMENT, K. I., KOENIG, H. G.; PEREZ, L. M. The many methods of religious coping: Development and initial validation of the RCOPE. **Journal of Clinical Psychology**. 2000. 56(4), 519-543.

PASKULIN, L. M. G. et al . Elderly people's perception of quality of life. **Acta paul. enferm.**, Sao Paulo , v. 23, n. 1, 2010 .

PENA, A. P. S.; GONCALVES, J. R. L. Assistência de enfermagem aos familiares cuidadores de alcoolistas. **SMAD, Rev. Eletrônica Saùde Mental Alcool Drog. (Ed. port.)**, Ribeirao Preto , v. 6, n. 1, 2010.

PENHA, R. M. **The expression of the spiritual dimension in ICU nursing care.** 2008. Dissertation (Master's Degree in Nursing in Adult Health) - School of Nursing, University of Sao Paulo, Sao Paulo, 2008.

PENHA, R.M.; SILVA, M. J. P. From Sensible to Intelligible: new directions in health communication through the study of Quantum Theory. **Revista da Escola de Enfermagem da USP**, v. 43, n. 1, p. 208-214, 2009.

PENHA, R. M. SILVA, Maria Jùlia Paes da. Meaning of spirituality for intensive care nursing. **Texto & Contexto Enfermagem**, v. 21, n. 2, p. 260, 2012.

PENROD, Janice et al. The influence of the culture of care on informal caregivers' experiences. **ANS. Advances in nursing science**, v. 35, n. 1, p. 64, 2012.

PEREIRA, M. J. S B.; FILGUEIRAS, M. S. T. Dependence in the aging process: a review on informal caregivers of the elderly. **Rev. APS**, Juiz de Fora, v. 12, n. 1, p. 72-82, 2009.

POULIN, M. J. et al. "Does a Helping Hand Mean a Heavy Heart? Helping Behavior and Well-Being Among Spouse Caregivers." **Psychology and aging** 25.1 (2010): 108-117. PMC.

PUCHALSKI, C. Task force report: spirituality, cultural issues, and end of life care. Assoc. of America Med. Colleg. Contemporary issues in medicine, communication in medicine.

Medical school objectives project. 1999.

PUCHALSKI C.; ROMER A. L. Taking a spiritual history allows clinicians to understand patients more fully. J Palliat Med 2000;3(1):129-37.

SALDANHA, R. C. M. Uso da rede de serviços de Juiz de Fora: a opinião dos utilizadores. In: **Revista Brasileira de Medicina de Familia e Comunidade**. v.4, n° 13, Rio de Janeiro, 2008.

SANCHES, I. M.; BOEMER, M. R. Living with pain: an existential approach. **Rev. Esc. Enferm. USP**, Sao Paulo, v. 36,n.4.

SANTOS, C.M. Self-care and educational process of elderly people with chronic non-communicable diseases who require nursing care at home. 2014. 153. Master's Degree in Nursing, Federal University of Juiz de Fora, Juiz de Fora.

SANTOS, F. K. How clients with chronic kidney disease cope with the onset of peritoneal dialysis: reflections on nursing care. **2009. Master's dissertation. Federal University of Rio de Janeiro. Anna Nery School of Nursing.**

SANTOS, S.M.A. Idosos, familia e cultura: um estudo sobre a construção do papel de cuidador. 3 ed. Campinas, SP: Alinea, 2010.

SARAIVA, K. R. O., et al. (2007). The process of living of the family caregiver in the adherence of the hypertensive user to treatment. **Texto e Contexto -enfermagem**, *16*(8), 63-70.

SEIMA, M. D; LENARDT, M. H; CALDAS, C. P. Relationship in care between the family caregiver and the elderly with Alzheimer's disease. **Revista Brasileira de Enfermagem**, v. 67, n. 2, p. 233, 2014.

SMEKE, E. L. M. Spirituality and primary health care: contributions to daily practice. In: VASCONCELOS, E. M. (Org.). **Spirituality in health work**. Sao Paulo: Hucitec, 2006.

SNODGRASS, J.; SORAJJAKOOL, S. Spirituality in older adulthood: Existential meaning, productivity, and life events. **Pastoral Psyciology**, v. 60, n. 1, p. 85-94, 2011.

SILVA, I. J. et al. Care, self-care and self-care: a paradigmatic understanding for nursing studies. **Rev. Esc. Enferm**. USP. v. 43, n. 3, p. 697-703, 2009.

SILVA, M. C.M.S. et al. Health education with the elderly: an experience report. **Rev. Raizes e Rumos.** UNIRIO. v. 2, n.2, 2014.

SOARES, S. M.; SILVA, L. B.; SILVA, P. A. B. O teatro em foco: estratégia lùdica para o trabalho educativo na saù da família. **Esc. Anna Nery**, Rio de Janeiro , v. 15, n. 4, Dec. 2011 .

SOUZA I.R., CALDAS C.P. Gerontological home care: contributions to the care of the elderly in the community. RBPS, v.21, n.1, p.61- 68, 2008.

SOUZA, R.B. What is spirituality? The biblical challenge of Christian spirituality. IN: BOMILCAR, N. (Org.). **O melior da espiritualidade brasileira.** Sao Paulo: Mundo Cristao, 2005. p. 13-33.

STARFIELD B. Primary care: balancing health needs, services and technology. Brasilia: UNESCO/Ministry of Health; 2004.

STRAUSS, A.; CORBIN, J. Bases de la Investigación Cualitativa: técnicas y procedimientos para desarrollar la teoria fundamentada. Antioquia: Universidad de Antioquia, 2002. Translated by Eva Zimmerman.

STRAUSS, A.; CORBIN, J. **Qualitative research: techniques and procedures for developing grounded theory.** 2ª ed. Porto Alegre: Artmed, 2008.

STRAUSS, A. Qualitative Analysis for Social Scientists. Cambridge (United Kingdom): University of Cambridge Press, 1987.

STROPPA, A.; MOREIRA-ALMEIDA, A. **Religiosidade e Saùde.** Chapter Published in: Saúde e Espiritualidade: uma nova vista da medicina Mauro Ivan Salgado & Gilson Freire (Orgs.).Belo Horizonte: Inede, 2008. (pp.: 427-443)

STREUBERT, H. J.; CARPENTER, D. R. **Qualitative research in nursing**: advancing the humanistic imperative. 2.ed. Philadelphia: Lippincott, p. 99-115, 1999.

SZYMANSKI, H. **Um estudo sobre significado de familia**. Sao Paulo: Pontifical Catholic University, 1992.

SZYMASNKI, H. Family life as an experience of mutual care. Serviço Social e Sociedade, Sao Paulo: Cortez, n.71, Sept. 2002.

TANYI, R. A. Towards clarification of the meaning of spirituality. **Journal of advanced nursing**, v. 39, n. 5, p. 500-509, 2002.

TEIXEIRA, M.Z. The nature of man: a comparative study of homeopathic vitalism with the main medical and philosophical conceptions. 2.ª ed. Sao Paulo: Marcus Zulin Teixeira, 2013.

TORNSTAM, L. **Gerotranscendence: A reformulation of the disengagement theory Aging**. 1, 55-63, 1989.

TORNSTAM, L. **Gerotranscendence: The contemplative dimension of aging.** 1997.

TURATO, E.R. Qualitative and quantitative methods in health: definitions, differences and their research objects. **Rev. Saùde Pùblica,** v. 39, 2005.

UNITED NATIONS. **Population Ageing and Development 2012.** New York, N.Y.:

Population Division, Department of Economic and Social Affairs, United Nations, 2012.

. **Basics Facts about the United Nations**. 2014. Published by the United

Nations Department of Public Information New York, New York 10017, United States of America. Revised Edition. ISBN: 978-92-1-056166-2.

FEDERAL UNIVERSITY OF JUIZ DE FORA. Social Research Center. **Socio-economic diagnosis of the elderly population of Juiz de Fora: profile of the elderly living in the urban area of Juiz de Fora**. Juiz de Fora: Extension Office, 2012.

VALLE, E. Conversão: da notão teòrica ao instrumento de pesquisa. 2002. **Revista de Estudos da Religiao**, Sao Paulo, N° 2: 51-76.

VASCONCELOS, A. M. N. ; GOMES, M. M. F. Demographic transition: the Brazilian experience. 2012.

VASCONCELOS, E. M. (org.). Spirituality in Health Work. Sao Paulo, Editora, Hucitec, 2006.

VERAS, R. P.; CALDAS, C. P. **UnATI-UERJ**: 10 years a model of comprehensive care for the ageing population. Rio de Janeiro: UnATI, 2004.

ViCTORA, C. G.; KNAUTH, D. R.; HASSEN, M. N. A. **Qualitative research in health:** an introduction to the theme. Porto Alegre: Tomo Editorial, 2000. p: 62-4.

VIEIRA, C.P.B. et al . Practices of the informal caregiver of the elderly at home. **Rev. bras. enferm.**, Brasilia , v. 64, n. 3, June 2011 .

WAHEY, L. F; WONG, D. L. **Enfermagem Pediàtrica**, Ed. Guanabara, Rio de Janeiro, 1989.

WALDOW, V. ; LOPES, M.; MEYER, D. - *Maneiras de cuidar, maneiras de ensinar: a enfermagem entre a escola e a prática profissional.* Porto Alegre: Artes Médicas, 1995. ISBN 85-7307-060-9.

WALDOW, V. R.; BORGES, R. F. Caring and humanizing: relationships and meanings. **Acta paul. enferm.**, Sao Paulo , v. 24, n. 3, 2011 .

WALSH, F. Fortalecendo a resiliência familiar. (M. F. Lopes, Trad.) Sao Paulo: Roca. 2005. (Original published in 1998).

WATSON, J. - *Enfermagem: ciência humana e cuidar - uma teoria de enfermagem.* Loures: Lusociência, 2002. ISBN 972-8383-33-9.

WORLD HEALTH ORGANIZATION. Geneva. **The uses of epidemiology in the study of the elderly**. Geneva: WHO, HEE 82.6Rev.11(3.87). Technical Report Series, 706, 1984.

10. APPENDIX

APPENDIX A

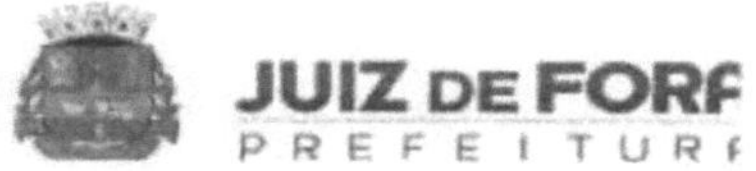

DECLARATION OF INTENT AND AGREEMENT

We authorize the research "Self-care of Elderly People Who Care for a Dependent Elderly Family Member at Home", to be conducted under the supervision of Prof. Edna Aparecida Barbosa de Castro (Faculty of NursingZUFJF) and her advisee Monalisa Claudia Maria da Silva Novaes.

The study will be carried out in Primary Health Care Units that work with the Family Health Strategy.

These facilities have the necessary infrastructure to carry out the research, which will only be able to begin field collection after the favorable opinion of the ZUFJF Research Ethics Committee has been presented to the Department for the Development of Primary Health Care of the Undersecretariat for Primary Health Care/ZPJF Health Department.

Juiz de Fora. February 20, 2014

Claudia Rocha Franco

Head of the Primary Health Care Department

APPENDIX B

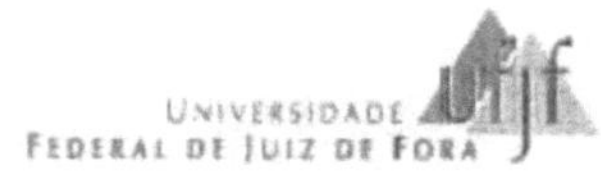

FACULDADE DE ENFERMAGEM

Profª Dr^a Girlene Alves da Silva
Prof^a. Dra. Girlene Alves da Silva
DIRETORA DA FACULDADE
DE ENFERMAGEM/UFJF

APPENDIX C

FRONT

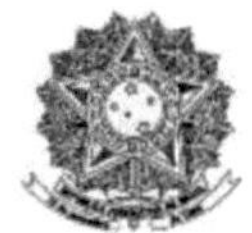

FEDERAL UNIVERSITY OF JUIZ DE FORA

RESEARCH ETHICS COMMITTEE - CEP HU/UFJF

JUIZ DE FORA - MG - BRAZIL

NAME OF RESEARCHER: FACULDADE DE ENFERMAGEM DA UNIVERSIDADE FEDERAL DE JUIZ DE FORA - RESPONSIBLE RESEARCHER: Professor Monalisa Claudia Maria da Silva Novaes - Master's student in Nursing - ADDRESS: RUA DIAS GOUVEIA, 16 B. BENFICA/ CEP: 36090-130 - JUIZ DE FORA - MG FONE(32) 3222-1264 - E- MAIL:monalisacms13@gmail. com E Professor Dra.^a Edna Aparecida Barbosa de Castro - ADDRESS: RUA HEITOR VILLA LOBOS, N° 11 - RESIDENCIAL SAO LUCAS I / SAO PEDRO. CEP: 36036-635 JUIZ DE FORA - MG PHONE: (32) 32311391 - E-MAIL: edna.catro@ujfj.edu.br

INFORMED CONSENT FORM

You are being invited as a volunteer to take part in the study **"Self-care of elderly people caring for an elderly relative at home"**. In this research we intend to understand how the self-care of elderly people who care for a dependent elderly relative at home takes place at the interface of the ESF nurse's work process and the SUS Home Care Policy. The reason for studying the self-care of the elderly caregiver is the aging trend of the Brazilian population, leading to a significant increase in the number of chronic-degenerative diseases and, with this, an increase in caregivers who are also elderly. In this study, the researcher will make home visits which will be scheduled according to the availability and acceptance of the elderly person. During these visits, the researcher will observe the life context of the elderly caregivers and will record in a diary only what is relevant to the research. An interview will be conducted according to a guiding script, which will be recorded and then listened to and transcribed in order to identify the most important information. The content of the interviews and observation notes will be used exclusively for academic and scientific purposes and will be archived by the research coordinator for five years, after which time they will be destroyed. The risk of participation is considered to be minimal, i.e. the same risk that exists in routine activities such as talking, reading, etc. The

167

researchers are concerned and careful to minimize these risks as much as possible with anonymity techniques, communication techniques, interpersonal interaction and human respect, with a non-interventionist approach. The benefits of carrying out this research include: Providing support for the nursing care process for elderly caregivers and instigating health policies so that the caregiver receives attention and support to carry out daily activities during visits by the health team, with quality guidance, in a resolutive and humanized way, in a structured family environment.

In order to take part in this survey, Mr. (a):

Your participation will be voluntary, at no cost to you and you will not receive any financial benefit;

S You will be informed about the study in any way you wish

S You are free to participate or refuse to participate, and you can withdraw your consent or stop participating at any time.

Refusal to participate will not lead to any penalty or change in the way you are treated by the researchers.

Your identity will be treated with professional standards of anonymity. You will not be identified in any publication that may result from this research. Your name or any material indicating your participation will not be released without your prior permission;

S You will have the right to compensation in the event that any damage caused by the research is proven, and this research presents minimal risk.

You will have the results of the survey at your disposal when it is finished.

This consent form is printed in two copies, one of which will be kept by the researcher in charge and the other will be given to you. I, ____________, bearing my identity document, have _ been informed of the objectives of the study **"Self-care of elderly people who**

care for an elderly relative at home" in a clear and detailed manner and I have clarified my doubts. I know that I can ask for further information at any time and change my decision to take part if I so wish. I declare that I agree to take part in this study. I have received a copy of this informed consent form and have been given the opportunity to read it and clarify my doubts.

Juiz de Fora, ____________________2014__________________________ .

Name	Participant signature	Date
Name	Signature of researcher	Date
Name	Witness signature	Date

If you have any questions about the ethical aspects of this study, you can consult the HU RESEARCH ETHICS COMMITTEE. HOSPITAL UNIVERSITARIO UNIDADE SANTA CATARINA - PREDIO DA ADMINISTRAÇÂO SALA 27. ZIP CODE 36036-110. E-mail: cep.hu@ufjf.edu.br

APPENDIX D - Semi-structured interview script.

RESEARCHER: Monalisa Claudia Maria da Silva

IDENTIFICATION:

Initials: _____________________ .

Date the questionnaire was administered:.

Age:

Sex:

Degree of kinship: _____________________

Education: _____________________________

Hά how long you've been a caregiver:

Guiding questions for the interview

1. Tell me how you started looking after your elderly relative?

2. What is it like for you to have to look after an elderly relative?

3. What difficulties do you experience when caring for your relative? How easy is it?

4. Do you receive help from other family members? From whom? How many times a week?

5. Do you feel safe when you are carrying out your day-to-day care activities?

6. What has changed in your life since you took on responsibility for your family member's care?

7. How do you take care of your own health?

8. How do you find relief from the stresses of everyday life?

9. What do you think could be done to improve your health? And who could do it?

10. Do you receive any information or support on a daily basis about how to care for your family member at home? From whom? From where?

11. Is the information and support you receive on a daily basis enough to facilitate your daily work process?

12. Anything else you'd like to say?

11. ANNEXES

ANNEX A - Consubstantiated Opinion Brazil Platform

UNIVERSITY HOSPITAL OF FEDERAL UNIVERSITY OFJUIZ DE FORA-MG

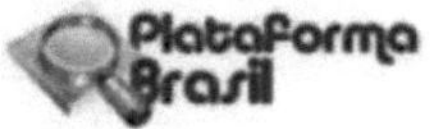

RESEARCH PROJECT DATA

Research title: Self-care of elderly people caring for a dependent elderly relative at home

Researcher: Monalisa Claudia Maria da silva

Thematic Area:

Version: 1

CAAE: 30978414.3.0000.5133

Proposing Institution: FEDERAL UNIVERSITY OF JUIZ DE FORA UFJF

Main Sponsor: Self-financing

OPINION DATA

Opinion Number: 676.364

Reporting date: 26/05/2014

Project presentation:

This qualitative study focuses on the self-care of elderly people who are caregivers for a dependent elderly relative. The emphasis will be on the support and education needs of the elderly, who care for the elderly, especially those that can be resolved in the context of the work process of nurses from the Family Health Strategy, when carrying out home care activities.

Research Objective:

Primary Objective: To understand the self-care of elderly people who care for a dependent elderly relative at home in the interface between the work process of the ESF nurse and the Home Care Policy in the SUS.

Secondary Objective: To analyze how elderly people who care for a dependent elderly relative care for themselves. To capture the facilities and difficulties of the elderly caregiver in the daily care of their elderly family member. To identify the sources of information and support for these elderly caregivers in their process of caring for their dependent family member at home. To develop a theoretical flowchart on the process of care at home by elderly caregivers of a dependent elderly family member.

Evaluation of Risks and Benefits:

Continuation of Opinion: 676.364

The risk of the subjects taking part in this research is considered to be minimal, i.e. similar to everyday life situations, and the researchers are concerned and attentive to minimizing these risks as much as possible with anonymity techniques, communication techniques and interaction techniques.

and human respect. It will also be able to provide support for the nursing care process for elderly caregivers and instigate health policies so that the caregiver receives attention and support to carry out daily activities during visits by the health team, with quality guidance, in a resolutive and humanized way, in a structured family environment.

Comments and Considerations on the Research:

The proposed study is pertinent and of scientific value, with a methodology suited to the objectives

clearly describing the methods used to collect and analyze the data. The inclusion and exclusion criteria are described, without compromising the vulnerability of the subjects, guaranteeing their right to information, privacy and withdrawal. The timetable is up to date.

Consideration of mandatory terms of presentation:

The mandatory terms were presented. The ICF does not make it clear that the research is of minimal risk and that, even so, the researcher will try to minimize them.

Recommendations:

Submit the report at the end of the research to the CEP

Conclusions or Pending Issues and List of Inadequacies:

Not applicable

Status of the opinion:

Approved

Needs CONEP appraisal:

No

Final considerations at the discretion of the CEP:

JUIZ DE FORA, June 05, 2014.

Signed by:
Gisele Aparecida Fófano
(Coordinator)

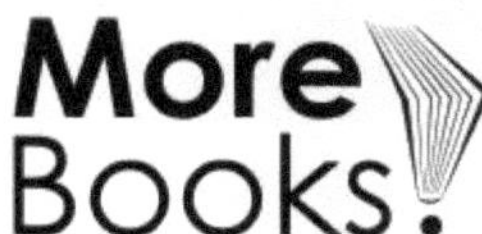
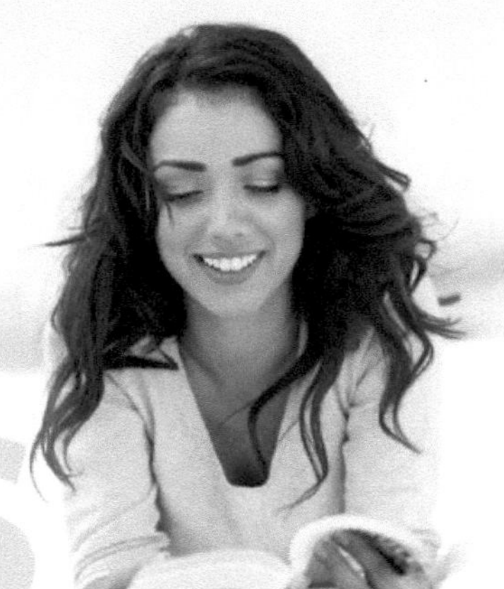

I want morebooks!

Buy your books fast and straightforward online - at one of world's fastest growing online book stores! Environmentally sound due to Print-on-Demand technologies.

Buy your books online at
www.morebooks.shop

Kaufen Sie Ihre Bücher schnell und unkompliziert online – auf einer der am schnellsten wachsenden Buchhandelsplattformen weltweit! Dank Print-On-Demand umwelt- und ressourcenschonend produziert.

Bücher schneller online kaufen
www.morebooks.shop

info@omniscriptum.com
www.omniscriptum.com

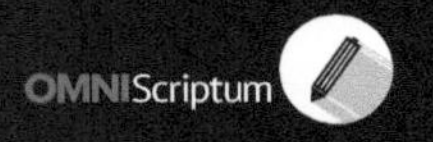

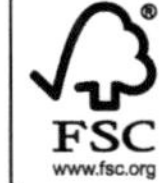

Printed by Books on Demand GmbH, Norderstedt / Germany